SELFISH

A Cardiologist's Guide to Healing a Broken Heart

Dr. Columbus Batiste

Heart Healthy Nation

PRAISE FOR AUTHOR

We must all embrace the kind of "Self*ish*" advocated by lifestyle medicine champion Dr. Columbus Batiste within the pages of this entertaining and enlightening book. Lifestyle medicine's six pillars include a whole food, plant-predominant dietary eating pattern, regular physical activity, restorative sleep, stress management, the avoidance of risky substances, and positive social connection that brings meaning and purpose to our lives. Let's follow Dr. Batiste's lifestyle medicine prescription to cure our stressed and broken hearts—it's what our world needs now!

- Susan Benigas
Executive Director, American College of Lifestyle Medicine

Dr. Columbus Batiste is one of the most caring, knowledgeable, and passionate doctors living today. His creation of the Self*ish* concept is a beautiful testament to his dedication to people living healthy and abundant lives. Reading his guide resonated with me because of my family's history with heart disease. This book gave me a true understanding and awareness of the impact of stress and broken- heartedness on our lives, and also gave me the permission needed to live my life with greater intentionality.

- Olivia F. Scott
Creator & Founder
Freedom At The Mat/ESSENCE Wellness House

Dr. Columbus Batiste, wearing his heart on his sleeve, walks us through his Self*ish* protocol to arm and insulate us against the #1 killer of men and women in this country: heart disease. Give this a read, protect your heart, and understand what it means to be Self*ish* in all the best ways!

- Rip Esselstyn
Founder & CEO, PLANTSTRONG Foods

In Self*ish* Dr. Batiste combines engaging stories, breakthrough research, and practical tips to help you live a more healthy and satisfying life. This is a comprehensive and holistic masterpiece that will lead the way to a brighter future. I encourage you to buy it, read it, and share it with everyone you love.

- Ocean Robbins
Co-founder, Food Revolution Network
Author, Real Superfoods

Dr. Columbus Batiste, M.D. skillfully navigates the reader through various forms of stress and lifestyle choices which can weaken and sometimes even destroy our health. Self*ish* is not just a book; it's a prescription for healing and resilience. Dr. Batiste's decades of experience as a double board-certified interventional cardiologist, shines through as he shares practical strategies for promoting mental and physical well-being. The book culminates in a powerful message: You are worth it, and by embracing the highly effective principles in this book, you can embark on a journey to transform your health.

- Chef AJ
Best-selling Author & Host of Chef AJ LIVE!

In a world saturated with divisive lifestyle approaches and desperate reductionism, filled with constant distractions that are only worsened by out-of-control, preventable diseases, Dr. Batiste's Self*ish* offers a perfect, step-by-step guide for optimum health and a happier, less stressful, more intentional life.

- Marco Borges
New York Times Best Selling Author & Exercise Physiologist

This empowering guide opens the door not only to a happier and more empowered life, but to a much healthier life as well. When maladaptive stress and less-than-healthy eating habits have you in their grip, this book presents a step-by-step guide to breaking free. Dr. Columbus Batiste is a leading cardiologist whose expertise has changed countless lives. This book will change yours as well.

Many are looking for natural healing and prevention with the "optimal" diet, exercise, and supplements, but they often overlook the power of spirituality and stress management as a core superpower. Dr. Columbus Batiste produces a masterpiece that focuses on the role of being Self*ish* in terms of self-care for the heart, the spirit, and the soul. A must-read for all my patients.

DEDICATION

From those seeking a path to genuine well-being to those who understand that "not everything that counts can be counted," this book is dedicated to the resilient hearts and curious minds ready to embark on the journey of Selfish transformation. May you find solace, wisdom, and lasting joy within these pages, guiding you toward a healthier, happier life.

- Dr. Columbus Batiste

CONTENTS

ACKNOWLEDGEMENT

IN THE TAPESTRY of my life, there are threads of gratitude woven into the intricate patterns of support and inspiration. To my life companion, my trusted confidante, the love of my life, my wife—your tough love and unwavering support has been the catalyst for my journey of growth. Instead of seeing achievements as endpoints, you've taught me to view them as commas, signaling that there is always more to explore and accomplish. Your encouragement has propelled me toward a greater purpose, and for that, I am eternally thankful.

To my father, whose passing created a void in my heart and instilled a lasting sense of guilt that has been a constant companion, shaping my purpose in life and guiding me onto the path of this wellness journey. You are the driving force behind my "why." Despite the deep longing to exchange this crusade for your continued presence, your memory serves as a powerful fuel for my pursuit. You remain a timeless inspiration, forever guiding my endeavors with your enduring influence.

To my mother, a living manifestation of love in action. Your sacrifices, spiritual guidance, and unwavering love for our family have profoundly influenced my perception of living with purpose, under- scoring the significance of anchoring every aspect of life in love. I am deeply appreciative of your inspiring example, in which you've showcased not only the power of love but also the essence of leading a purposeful and meaningful life.

To my son and daughter, you are profound sources of motivation. My greatest aspiration is to leave you the wisdom to lead mentally and physically healthy lives. Your capabilities are boundless, and I want you to understand that true fulfillment comes when achievements align with purpose. In giving me purpose, you have bestowed upon me the most meaningful gift. Thank you for inspiring me to guide you toward a purposeful and abundant life.

To my siblings, your steadfast examples and unwavering support have been both a compass and an anchor through challenging times. Thank you for being pillars of strength and sources of unwavering support. Together, we have weathered storms and celebrated triumphs, creating a tapestry of shared experiences that I cherish deeply.

In acknowledging each of you, I recognize that this journey is not solitary but a collective effort—a symphony of love, inspiration, and resilience that has shaped the pages of my life.

INTRODUCTION

Every compelling superhero movie unveils an origin story that reveals the journey they took to become heroes. This transformation often springs from tragedy, such as the loss of a loved one or confronting life-threatening situations. Regardless of the trigger, something within them ignites their latent greatness.

In Spiderman's origin story, Peter Parker was bitten by a genetically altered spider, gaining spider-like superpowers. However, his selfish choices prevented him from saving his Uncle Ben's life. Witnessing his father figure's death left him shattered, but he rose from grief, inspired by Ben's final lesson: "With great power comes great responsibility." He harnessed his superhuman abilities for the greater good, becoming a genuine superhero.

Batman's origin story showcases how Bruce Wayne transformed into the crime-fighting Dark Knight (Batman) after witnessing his parents' tragic death at the hands of a robber. In homage to them, he vowed to combat crime and rebuild the community that bred his parents' killers. What's remarkable about the Bruce Wayne transformation is that he didn't even have superpowers; his strength lay in his passion, purpose, and commitment to change his community. He converted his parents' tragedy into his life's mission.

I am an interventional cardiologist. I'm not a superhero, and I don't have superpowers, but I, too, have an origin story. Mine is a heartrending tale that altered my career trajectory and propelled me to a life of crime fighting. What does a doctor know about crime fighting? A lot. Crime fighting in some ways is synonymous with disease fighting because most of the chronic diseases we face today are akin to a preventable crime or unnecessary tragedy. My personal tragedy led me to see disease from a different vantage point and as a result, prompted a shift from just treating the aftermath of disease to preventing its occurrence through potent healing strategies.

Just like Spiderman and Batman, my origin story began with a tragic loss. In the afternoon of August 12, 2010, at 2:15 p.m., I watched my father die from the complications of diabetes. Besides the loss of a father, the tragedy is that his death didn't have to happen like that. Diabetes is mostly a preventable disease that often requires altering one's lifestyle; it was a crime that didn't have to happen. That trauma of watching my first role model, my dad, die, was devastating. Here I was, a triple board-certified interventional cardiologist —board certified in internal medicine, general cardiology, and interventional cardiology—and I didn't or couldn't save my own father. The irony is that throughout my career, I've been thanked countless times for saving patients' lives, but like Spiderman, I watched a crime occur that could have been stopped. That should have been stopped, but it wasn't. It wasn't a sudden death. If I'm honest, I watched my father die slowly, inch by inch, for years before the end. And I admit with great shame that I stood by and did nothing outside of encouraging the standard of care: pills and procedures. After his death, the guilt that I could have done more was overwhelming, and to this day, the memories still haunt me. The day my dad died was one of my darkest moments. I was plagued by "what if's. I ruminated over all the things I should have done. My mind replayed life events and the countless opportunities I had to intervene. Looking back, I think the stress from grief made my mind spiral. Or maybe my spiraling mind made me stressed. I'm not sure of the exact cause, but stress forcefully reared its head. Had it not been for the seeds of resiliency and hope my parents planted in me when I was growing up, I might still be spiraling in grief. The seeds of resiliency my parents planted sprouted and flourished and set me on a new course. So, like the phoenix, I arose from the ashes of depression and began to search my dad's life for a clue as to how I may have helped him.

I discovered the role that stress plays in both mental and physical disease. The significance and potency of exercise and rest in maintaining overall well-being became clear to me. I unearthed the power of spirituality, intimacy of relationships, love, and humor over perceived stress and their impact on physical health. In my exploration, I came to understand the dual nature of food; both its potential to bolster health and, conversely, contribute to disease. Through my research, I realized that the choices we make regarding our diet can either intensify our stress levels or enhance our capacity to endure it. This insight prompted me to introduce the terms *"nutritional stress"* and *"nutritional resiliency."* The more I grasped these concepts, the more perplexed I became about the absence of this knowledge in my medical training. Despite being a board-certified physician, my formal education had failed to equip me to holistically care for my patients.

As I reflected on my journey, I began to wonder if my inaction during my father's health battle was unconsciously influenced by the deep-seated belief that chronic diseases like diabetes and heart disease are simply our destiny, which immobilized me. Regardless, his passing was a wake-up call for me. It made me realize that the reductionist model I was taught in training, which focused on isolated mechanisms of disease and health, was inadequate. True health is an intricate interplay of various aspects of life, a realization that dawned on me through introspection.

After rigorous self-education, I was armed with new tools. I felt complete for the first time as a physician. At last, I was able to holistically address the health of my patients and convince them that their DNA is not their destiny. Now, after more than a decade of applying these principles and developing lifestyle programs in my practice, it is time to share my prescription to cure a stressed and broken heart. If you take away one thing from this book, it should be that you are worth it. You deserve to live a healthy, purpose-filled life, but in order to do so, you will need to be Self*ish*. If you apply the Self*ish principles* in this book, you can promote healing in your mind and body that will allow you to live a healthy life and a life of purpose.

CHAPTER 1

What Is Stress?

In today's world, one of the buzzwords is "stress," and no wonder. Our lives are filled with demands that call for more than we are equipped to handle. What is stress? Each one of us probably has a definition, but I define stress as an internal reaction to external stimuli. When I was in training and just out of medical school, I remember being up all night. This was back in the days when, symbolically, you had to walk backward, up a hill, in the snow to become a board-certified physician. Once, I was up all night taking care of patients and running around fulfilling endless demands. I worked for 36 hours straight without sleep. There was no downtime. My sister called. I was exhausted, groggy, and irritable as I listened to what I thought was her inconsideration. She just didn't understand. "Columbus, did you take care of such-and-such for our parents?" How could she ask that of me?

"Do you understand how stressed I am?"

Her reply is permanently etched in my mind: "You're not the only one who is stressed. I have a young baby, and if I'm up all night and all day and I don't get sleep, there will be problems with the baby."

A light switched on in my mind as her words gave me a new understanding of stress.

> *Stress is a perception, and it's hard to equate a person's experience and their reaction to life's circumstances to what you're going through.*

A more clinical definition is that stress is a state of mental or emotional strain. It happens when you perceive life's demands are more than what you can handle with your own abilities or help from others. So, the more things you have to deal with and the less support you think you have, the more stressed you'll feel. There are actually two types of stress; one that can be good (eustress) and one that's not so good (distress). But when most of us think about stress, we usually think about the bad kind, so let's focus on the not-so-good stress, the distress. It's split into three categories: acute stress, which is short and intense, episodic stress, and chronic stress. Acute stress happens briefly. It might be when you almost get into a car accident, or when you have to finish a school project really quickly. It could even be something like being chased by a dog or jumping away from a snake. These situations trigger our bodies to release hormones like adrenaline and cortisol. Once the danger passes, the stress goes away. Episodic stress occurs when acute stress situations occur too often. People who take on too much are candidates for episodic stress. These two kinds of stress are pervasive across all species. Chronic stress is different. It's when stress lasts for a long time. This type of stress is more common in humans. It can happen if you have a really demanding job, ongoing money problems, or difficult relationships that don't get better.

Eustress is considered a positive stress. Eustress occurs when normal stress is felt as motivational to the individual. It can stimulate us to work toward our goals. Meeting realistic but sometimes difficult challenges can bring a sense of accomplishment and fulfillment. It occurs when people turn difficult situations into learning opportunities or choose to reframe negative situations into positive ones. It occurs when people feel confident in their ability to solve a problem or cope with the situation. Some call that a *challenge response*. A challenge response occurs when athletes perform under pressure. They make the point that wins the championship game, and the crowd goes wild while the player breathes a sigh of relief and feels happiness and pride. When students feel stressed about an upcoming test but they know that they are prepared, they celebrate when they know they have aced it. Eustress is like lifting weights to build muscles. It's not that easy to lift those weights, but doing so provides us with our desired results. Think ripped!

The Connection Between Stress and Health

The year 2020 affected everyone. The pandemic brought forth a kind of stress we had never dealt with before. From the elderly woman who was not allowed to go to the hospital and be with her dying husband, to the grocery store worker who was deemed a superhero, we were forced into a narrow lifestyle that frustrated many, desiccated businesses, and put millions temporarily out of work. Our social needs went out the window. No longer could we enjoy a leisurely lunch with our best friends. Children celebrated their birthdays with their friends riding by their homes holding up brightly colored celebratory signs.

The virus that triggered this chain of stressful events was later found to enter our bodies through a layer of cells in blood vessels known as the endothelium.

This tragic experience highlighted to medical professionals that the connection between stress and health lies in our endothelium. The word endothelium is tossed around frequently by cardiologists, but most people have never heard of it. You probably need to know a little about endothelium if you want to understand how stress affects your body. If you are not a Cardiologist, here's the simplified version: Vascular endothelium is the inner lining of the blood vessels. It's like the thin coating on the nonstick frying pan that prevents food from sticking and liquids from being absorbed. Similarly, endothelium protects blood vessels by preventing things from sticking, which means clotting, in our vessels. The endothelium is responsive to the body's needs. The endothelium can cause dilation, enlargement, constriction, or narrowing of our vessels. The endothelium causes our vessels to expand in hot environments or to contract when it's cold. Stress can influence the endothelium. Stress can trigger the vessels to constrict, and when the vessels are smaller, blood pressure goes up. You know that old, scratched frying pan in your kitchen cabinet, the one that no longer keeps your food from sticking? When we are stressed, the same phenomenon happens in our bodies. The endothelium can become damaged and lose its protective function. It would be like Superman losing his protection from the sun. When the endothelium is damaged, it becomes sticky, which promotes inflammation, like a pimple. Compromised endothelium becomes infiltrated by cholesterol and other invaders, which causes the vessels to become stiff and calcified with protruding plaques in the lumen-like stalactites hanging from the ceiling of a cave.

Although doctors don't check for endothelial function in their clinics, it's a simple test that utilizes a blood pressure cuff and an ultrasound machine. You may be familiar with the ultrasound machines they use in the movies to reveal a tender moment as the pregnant mother and father look at their baby before birth. Scientists and physicians can look at an artery using ultrasound technology to determine how much a vessel enlarges after it's been compressed. It's somewhat like a rubber garden hose. When you press it down and release it, it returns to its original shape. But an old rubber hose is stiff and does not compress or expand easily. In damaged arteries, the endothelium doesn't expand after being compressed (we call that flow-mediated dilatation, or FMD) as much as arteries with healthy, undamaged endothelium. This is a marker of disease, and believe it or not, is also caused by stress.

Research has identified chronic diseases like high blood pressure, diabetes, or high cholesterol as conditions that lead to endothelium damage. Smoking, eating junk food, and eating foods rich in saturated fats and oils that become solid when in normal temperatures can lead to endothelium damage as well. Medical studies show that stress, specifically distress, can cause and lead to endothelium damage. This is serious stuff because damage to the endothelium is associated with strokes, dementia, heart attacks, kidney disease, erectile dysfunction, and even broken heart syndrome. In 2020, researchers discovered that the SARS-CoV-2 virus can infiltrate and infect damaged endothelial cells. These cells served as the entry point for the virus, leading to infection with the SARS-CoV-2 virus. Further studies have confirmed that individuals with compromised endothelial cells are more likely to experience severe symptoms and dangerous events from COVID-19. This has brought to light the importance of the endothelium in maintaining overall health and its crucial role in the connection between stress and health.

Allostasis

Allostasis refers to how a body's physiologic system changes to meet the demands of the environment. This ability to adapt is essential. An allostatic load is the price people pay for adapting to stress. It's basically wear and tear. When faced with stress, the body responds in a variety of ways to help you cope with the threat, this is allostasis. This is similar to the concept of a broken heart. If you've constantly had your heart broken, you've had someone cheat on you, or someone close to you has betrayed your confidence and trust, you begin to build a wall. This wall keeps people at a distance so they can't hurt you. It protects you and allows you to cope with the stress and the impact of this relationship. Allostatic load is the wear and tear on the body which accumulates as one is exposed repeatedly to chronic stress. Allostatic load refers to the damage that stress can do to the body over time, while the physical reactions that stress creates play a role in protecting the body. In the short term, allostatic load can help the body adapt to challenges and survive, while over the long term, it contributes to an increased vulnerability to disease. Remember that wall one builds to protect one from a toxic relationship? It might be protective in the short term, but in other relationships, it keeps the person at a distance and doesn't allow them to have the meaningful connections that they truly desire.

The Relationship Between Stress and Disease

Health equals resiliency divided by stress. Simply put, the higher your stress, the poorer your health. Chuck Swindoll, pastor, author, educator, and radio preacher, says stress is 10% what happens to you and 90% how you respond. We just learned that allostatic load is the accumulation of how your body responds to stressors. Research shows that every system in the body can be influenced by chronic stress. When chronic stress goes unpoliced, it's like when your car is parked in the driveway and you're warming it up. You press on the accelerator, but the car is in park and the emergency brake is on. The system is revved up, prepared to go, but the energy created cannot be used because the car is in park. The car is not going anywhere, and the car is damaged. That's how it is with chronic stress: The body mobilizes for action but there is no action, and the body is injured. Chronic stress suppresses the body's immune system and ultimately manifests as illness. One such illness is asthma. Asthma is a chronic lung disease that affects the airways of people with this condition, causing the airways to become inflamed, narrowed, and filled with secretions. This makes breathing difficult. Studies show that when people feel social stress, it can make the inflammation caused by allergens in asthma last longer. This can make asthma attacks happen more often and lead to more asthma-related sickness and even death. Scientists have found that stress can change how certain cells in our body, like airway cells, respond to corticosteroids, which are medicines used to treat asthma. This change can make immune cells work more, making asthma worse. The impact of stress in asthma flare-ups is why family therapy is widely incorporated in families that have asthmatic children. In addition to standard treatments, it is important to address the emotional and psychological stress that may contribute to asthma.   I had asthma when I was a child. If there was an argument, my asthma acted up. But to be honest, I may have faked an asthma attack or two to get out of trouble. Okay, I never said I was perfect. Let's label that as creative—or perhaps ingenious.

In addition to asthma, other illnesses, like gastrointestinal diseases, peptic ulcer disease, and ulcerative colitis, are influenced by stress. Data suggests that air traffic controllers have a more stressful job than civilian co-pilots. Peptic ulcer disease occurs twice as often in air traffic controllers than in civilian copilots. Peptic ulcer disease occurs more often among air traffic controllers who work in high stress centers like Dallas-Fort Worth, Chicago O'Hare, and the Los Angeles Airport than in those who work in low stress airports like Wichita, Huntsville, Asheville, Birmingham, and Tulsa inferring the direct relationship between stress levels and peptic ulcer disease. Ulcers are often caused by excessive stomach acid, and studies of patients with gastric fistulas reveal that anger and hostility increase your stomach acidity, while depression and withdrawal decrease acidity. Another theory of the development of peptic ulcer disease states that during chronic stress, your adrenaline secretion, one of the hormones that communicates with the body, causes the capillaries (refined blood vessels in the stomach lining) to constrict. This narrowing results in shutting down the mucosal production; therefore, the mucus protective barrier in the stomach is lost. Without that protective barrier, the acid in the stomach breaks down the tissue and can cause an ulcer. If the acid reaches the blood vessels, it results in a bleeding ulcer.

Enough about the lungs and the stomach system, my specialty is the heart. I literally see the effects of stress on the hearts of my patients daily. To excuse the pun, it is heartbreaking. There are many studies that show the effects of stress on the heart. The Interheart Study revealed that people with heart attacks reported higher levels of four stress factors: stress at work, stress at home, financial stress, and major life events within the past year. Additional studies show that heightened activity in the amygdala, that portion of the brain that stores fear memories, was linked to increased bone marrow activity, inflammation in the arteries, and a higher risk of heart attack and other cardiovascular events. To summarize, the higher the activity in the amygdala, the greater the likelihood of heart-related events.

It is abundantly clear that stress is related to disease. Stress doesn't just affect asthma and the development of ulcers and heart disease. Studies have shown that the increased levels of stress are predictive of Alzheimer's disease, high blood pressure, diabetes, and cancer. Our health equals resiliency divided by stress.

Angie's Story

I first met Angie in 2020. She was referred to me because she had chest pains. Unlike the past, when I could see my patients face to face, Angie came to me during the 2020 pandemic. That was the year the world changed. I am sure you were impacted, and just as you had to change your lifestyle, the medical profession was forced to change as well. I was still trying to figure out how to be a doctor in a virtual world. Angie and I both fumbled as we tried to replicate a face-to-face visit over the telephone. During that first visit, I could tell she was emotional, and I knew a telephone call was not enough. I usually didn't make video calls, nor would I interrupt a visit, but it was necessary. I asked her, "Are you willing to do this by video? I really feel this conversation should be as close to face-to-face as possible." She was willing, and we connected.

It is said there are five forms of communication: verbal communication, nonverbal communication, written communication, visual communication, and listening. The addition of visual and non-verbal communication the video provided created an emotional connection as I listened to her share her grief. She talked about the fear she experienced not knowing what was happening to her mother when she was admitted to the hospital during the pandemic. She described the guilt from not being able to visit her mom or hold her hand as she passed away. Since her mother's death, Angie recounted having recurring nightmares of her mom dying alone and the challenges of grieving by herself, with the Coronavirus preventing family gatherings.

Angie was worn down, and as she told her story, tears streamed down her face. She was at the end of her proverbial rope. She needed someone to talk to, and I felt I needed to listen. She told me that her symptoms had started when the family was not able to commemorate her mother's passing in their cultural tradition. When the pain began, she started experiencing tightness inside her chest that traveled to her jaw. She also experienced shortness of breath. She suffered sleepless nights, and she began to console herself with food. She felt depressed, but she was a mother who home-schooled her children, so she did not have the luxury of losing it, nor could she take the time to process her emotions. She was also a businesswoman who had to put on a professional front. She had to be strong for everyone. During this time, as if she did not have enough to deal with, she started having marital difficulties. The constraints of isolation and the pandemic put an extra burden on all aspects of her life, including her relationship with her husband. She told me she had an argument with her husband just the night before our consultation which triggered the pain. She described the pain as unbearable, and it kept her from sleeping. As she recalled the latest episode, she began to experience the symptoms again. I could see the pain on her face as she grimaced. It was so bad, she spoke in broken sentences and gasped for air. She was sweating, and I became increasingly alarmed.

"You need to go to the emergency room now!"

She looked at me with astonishment. "I'm not going to the hospital and getting exposed to that virus. My mama died of that disease, and I'm not going." I told her it was imperative and that we needed to call 911. I was worried, concerned that she might not live another day to take care of her children. From the monitor, I could see her children stood around her, anxious as they watched her crying and in pain.

I finally convinced her to call 911 and stayed on the phone with her until the ambulance arrived. I met her in the emergency room. We started our workup and quickly found her electrocardiogram results and her blood work were abnormal. We tested for COVID and fortunately, she was negative, but her test results pointed to an impending heart attack. Given her progressive symptoms and abnormal testing to that point, I recommended Angie undergo a cardiac catheterization. Cardiac catheterization is a medical procedure used to diagnose and treat conditions affecting the heart and blood vessels. During the procedure, a thin, flexible tube called a catheter is inserted into a blood vessel and guided to the heart.

We performed the cardiac catheterization procedure, which allowed us to look for blockages in her vessels. To my surprise, we found no blockages. We moved on to test her heart function. Was her heart able to squeeze out an adequate amount of blood? A normal heart is able to squeeze out about two thirds of the blood, or 65%. As we observed Angie's heart, what we saw astonished us. Her heart was paralyzed, it was moving outward instead of inward, and the heart function was severely reduced. Angie had a condition called Broken Heart Syndrome.

Broken Heart Syndrome

Broken Heart Syndrome, also referred to as Takotsubo Syndrome, or stress-induced cardiomyopathy, is a medical phenomenon characterized by an unusual condition in which the left ventricle, the heart's bottom pumping chamber, balloons outwardly instead of squeezing inwardly during periods of acute stress. Often triggered by intense emotions such as fear or anxiety, this condition can also be induced by various stressors, including relationship and financial concerns.

The recognition of Broken Heart Syndrome emerged in 1990 in Japan, initially termed "takotsubo" due to its resemblance to a traditional octopus trapping pot used by fishermen. This pot is characterized by a narrow neck and a broad, rounded base. The choice of the term "takotsubo" was due to its visual similarity to the weakened shape of the heart's left ventricle, as observed through medical imaging techniques like echocardiograms.

This condition disproportionately affects postmenopausal women, constituting approximately 90% of cases. The elevated prevalence of Broken Heart Syndrome among women compared to men raises the question of why, since both genders experience stress. One prevailing theory suggests that the decline in estrogen levels associated with postmenopausal changes renders women more susceptible. Decreasing estrogen levels, known to shield the heart from the detrimental impacts of stress hormones, potentially places women at greater risk.

Typical symptoms of Broken Heart Syndrome include chest discomfort, breathlessness, dizziness, weakness, and occasional fainting, mirroring those of a heart attack. Notably, Angie, as a case example, exhibited these symptoms. Since the symptoms resemble those of a heart attack, physicians frequently perform a safe but invasive procedure called cardiac catheterization to visualize the patient's coronary arteries. As in Angie's case, individuals with Broken Heart Syndrome typically lack such blockages.

So, how does the heart become paralyzed? The answer is a six-letter word: STRESS. More specifically, the body's response to stress (allostasis) through stress hormone production. Stress hormones underlie this heart condition and contribute to the temporary paralysis of the heart muscle by affecting the heart's blood vessels. This hormonal influence can disrupt the heart's normal function, leading to the ballooning of the left ventricle instead of its usual contraction.

For a deeper understanding, let's look at the amygdala. It is a portion of your brain that stores all of your history, including all fears, stress, and anxiety. Though the amygdala is small, it is powerful and can have a great impact on our bodies. The amygdala is responsible for processing and expressing emotions, especially anger and fear. It is always on the lookout for danger or times when we feel threatened.

When I was a kid, I watched the movie *Ben*, which portrayed rats running all over the place attacking people. From that moment on, I was terrified and anxious whenever I saw any rodent! This event was stored in my amygdala, and that memory resurfaces and triggers the same emotions and fears I had while watching the movie. Now, every time I see a rodent, I might jump on a table or chair (if I'm not in public; I do have my pride). When the amygdala senses danger, it can override reason and take over. This response allows us to act before we think. This reaction can be useful in a crisis, but the problem is that a chronically stressed amygdala can prime the heart to overreact during an acute stressful event. We see this happen repeatedly. A 2021 research study demonstrated that people who had higher activity in the amygdala, determined through a magnetic resonance imaging (MRI) study, had increased occurrences of Broken Heart Syndrome. This study of the amygdala led researchers to conclude that this syndrome happens because of chronic stress. Ongoing long-term stress predisposes people to develop Broken Heart Syndrome, and people with less stress are less likely to develop the syndrome.

More on Stress

Let's simplify the conversation on stress and divide stress into two categories—eustress and distress. Distress, as I mentioned before, is divided into three categories, but for now, we will put them all in one category. For concrete examples of distress, think about a student who does not study for an upcoming exam. They will probably feel panicked. Or a team player who has not practiced and misses a shot. They will probably feel guilty because they know they should have practiced. Stress can be simplified into an equation: Stress equals demands minus resources. When an individual's demands of life exceed their real or perceived resources, stress ensues. When you make $2,400 a month and your bills are $3,000 a month, you will feel stressed because your demands are higher than your resources. Remember Angie? Her emotional demands exceeded her ability to cope, and she felt out of control.

Another hidden form of stress is discrimination and bias. Discrimination exposes us to an increased stress response. One of my colleagues of Asian descent told the following story:

"At the end of the pandemic, I was walking through the hospital and encountered a man in the coffee line. He asked if I was Chinese. I told him I was not, but he continued to ask if I was Chinese and proceeded to inform me that the Chinese caused the pandemic. I felt attacked. Now, when I walk with my children and people stare, I worry, wondering if the stare will lead to a confrontation. I am triggered."

Once again, that amygdala response of fear and anxiety triggered the stress hormone, which then flowed throughout her body. Suppose you are a member of a religious group whose church is bombed. Will you be triggered when you return to church? You may even have post-traumatic stress disorder. This kind of stress or distress dismantles your entire life. In communities with a high level of frisking, researchers found increased levels of PTSD, nervousness, and mental stress, *not only in those touched directly by the law system but also in others within the community*. This means if an individual sees something traumatic or distressing happen to someone they associate with, they may experience, by proxy, increased stress.

Stress can trigger our "fight or flight" response. This response prepares us to engage or to run away and is triggered by a release of hormones called catecholamines and glucocorticoids. These are specialized names, but hormones are basically messengers that send signals telling our bodies' systems how to react. The message might tell the body it's time to attack, or that it's time to flee. When you see a lion coming toward you and he looks hungry or angry, it's time to flee. If your house catches on fire, you will want to flee. If a dog attacks your child, you will want to fight. This response serves an essential role in the short term because it prepares us to deal with threats, but it is harmful to be in this mode all the time. When we feel threatened, the body's physiological strategy is to increase our heart and breathing rates, tighten our muscles, and prepare the muscles for action by feeding them sugar released from the liver. Our blood pressure rises as our blood vessels clamp down. This creates a hypertensive state. Even our vision shifts as we prepare for action. When this repetitive stress response continues over long periods of time, it can cause physical damage.

The Superwoman Schema

The Superwoman Schema is a concept deeply rooted in research within the African American community, representing the epitome of allostasis in practice. It involves a mindset that some people, particularly African American women, adopt, akin to having a mental checklist of being a "superwoman" who can handle everything perfectly. This might entail striving for excellence in work, taking care of family, and confronting challenges like discrimination without displaying any signs of struggle. It's like feeling the constant pressure to be superhuman; perpetually strong and capable, even when it's not realistic.

This belief system imposes the notion that women must excel and flawlessly fulfill every role they undertake without revealing any vulnerabilities or shortcomings. Consequently, the relentless pursuit of this unattainable benchmark leads to chronic stress and burnout. The Superwoman Schema has been developed based on extensive studies focused on African American women from diverse age groups, affiliations, and educational backgrounds. These studies aim to gain insights into how African American women navigate and manage the manifold stresses of life, including discrimination, parenting, and inequalities, unveiling a recurring pattern characterized by its exceedingly demanding nature.

Researchers have identified a set of five defining characteristics that encapsulate the superwoman schema:

- Feeling a perceived obligation to project strength.

- Feeling a perceived obligation to suppress their emotions due to the fear of appearing weak.

- Feeling a perceived obligation to resist help or being vulnerable to others.

- Being motivated to succeed despite limited resources, adverse circumstances, or unequal resource distribution.

- Prioritizing caregiving over self-care.

It's important to remember the concepts of allostasis and allostatic load. Just like in ANGIE's story, who experienced the negative consequences of being a superwoman, too much of a good thing can harm one's health in the long run. A 2019 study also revealed that adopting a superwoman schema is linked to risk factors that can make women more susceptible to health problems, including heart disease.

Where Stress and Health Intersect

When we last talked about Angie's journey, I had just diagnosed her with something called Broken Heart Syndrome. This is when your heart doesn't work well because of all the stress you're going through.

But, over time, Angie bounced back and got her strength back. She lost some weight, felt more energetic, and saw life in a new way. Everything seemed to be getting better. Her heart was working better, and her blood pressure and markers for diabetes had improved as well. So, we set up a face-to-face appointment for a follow-up six months later.

You might remember that Angie first came to me during the pandemic in 2020-2021 when we couldn't have regular in-person doctor's visits, so we had to use phones and video calls. When we finally scheduled an in-person visit after almost nine months, I was really excited to see how she was doing after all those virtual appointments during the pandemic.

But when I walked into the exam room, my excitement faded. Angie had gained back the weight she'd lost and was even heavier. Her blood pressure and markers for diabetes were too high. She told me that the only time she had for herself was late at night, after work and taking care of everyone else. That was when she could relax, usually with her favorite comfort food. She talked about how the pandemic had affected her personal relationships. She said that after years of homeschooling her kids, they had moved on to the next part of their lives and didn't live at home anymore. She now felt a deep void. This sadness was made even worse because she was still grieving the loss of her mother. On top of all this, her husband had asked for a divorce after being married for 30 years, which amplified her sadness and loneliness. Angie was in tears as she told me that she felt like her heart had broken all over again, but in a different way. My joy in her previous success quickly vanished as I witnessed her pain and struggle.

I recognized that I hadn't helped her address the root cause of her pain. I realized that the pills, procedures, and gentle encouragement were not enough to give her the tools and resiliency she needed to combat the inevitable stressors of life. Instead of offering physical comfort, I spoke sternly to Angie and told her that she needed to learn to get "Self*ish*." I could see that my words had triggered an emotional response, leaving her silent and staring at me. I emphasized that her health and relationship issues were a result of her neglecting herself. I told her that she needed to make herself a priority. I explained the benefits of being Self*ish* and the power of resiliency in rebuilding her mental and physical health.

The thoughts I shared with Angie are concepts that are relevant to everyone's health. Self*ish* doesn't mean what most people think it means. Although being selfish is defined as concern with one's own welfare or advantage in disregard of others, getting Self*ish* is about developing a skillset and the habits that will allow you to achieve the health you deserve and live a life of purpose.

Self*ish* isn't just about your body. Turning Self*ish* into an acronym, the first **"S" stands for Spiritual.** The essence of Self*ish* starts with getting Spiritual. Spirituality, which comes from the Latin term spiritus meaning breath, is all about the connection that people have with God. It is influenced by cultural traditions, religious practices, and upbringing. Spirituality provides comfort for people, whether they draw from childhood traditions or embrace new ones. It becomes a valuable resource for those who are dealing with stress and chronic diseases. Spirituality is a means of feeding your soul—feeding who you are at the deepest level. Self*ish* spirituality is about connection, focus, and transformation through meditation, prayer, or thoughtful reflection. It also includes conscious breathing techniques. Cultivating habits that deeply support health, such as these spiritual practices, serves as key cornerstone habits, empowering individuals to enact desired changes in their lives and combat stress effectively.

For the next letter, *"E" stands for Exercise.* Exercise or movement helps us reduce stress, and as we reduce our stress levels, we reduce anxiety and depression. That is the power of exercise. It supercharges our metabolism, it empowers our immune system, and it fights against chronic disease.

Back to our acronym, S-E-L-F-I-S-H. The *"L" in* **Selfish** *stands for Love.*

> *"Love cannot exist in isolation; it derives its meaning from action." - Mother Teresa*

The actions or expressions of love include gratitude, forgiveness, and the act of selflessness. These elements hold significant value within relationships and serve as vital components when dealing with stress or healing a broken heart.

The *"F" in* **Selfish** *stands for Food,* *real* food—whole, plant-rich food, fiber-filled food, resilient food that nourishes the mind, body, and soul. Nourishment that adds to one's resiliency and has the potential to decrease the burden of stress and the power to send chronic disease into remission.

The *"I"* *in* **Selfish** *stands for Intimacy,* or meaningful relationships. They can be with a pet, a friend, your spouse, or with a lover. In intimate and trusting relationships, you can lower your emotional wall and be vulnerable. Vulnerability strengthens us. Studies show that intimate relationships are health-promoting. They can reduce the burden of perceived stress.

The second *"S"* *in the* **Selfish** *concept represents Sleep*, a profoundly underrated yet potent element that fuels improved self-control and initiates the healing process. Achieving sufficient sleep, coupled with intervals of rest, relaxation, and dedicated personal time or vacations, assumes a critical role in optimizing our mental and physical well-being. This practice not only alleviates the burden of stress but also spearheads the fight against chronic diseases and heart health.

The *"H" in* **Selfish** *represents Humor*, symbolizing joy and laughter. The age-old saying that laughter is the best medicine isn't just a cliché, it holds true in the scientific realm. Joy and laughter possess the remarkable power to mend the heart and rejuvenate the spirit, empowering you to cultivate the resilience necessary to alleviate the weight of stress and disease.

Each pillar in the Self*ish* principle has been independently shown to reduce one's perception of stress, reduce the heightened stress response, and restore the critical link between stress and health, known as the endothelium. My patient Angie's experience was not unique. I suspect you may have experienced challenges in your efforts to obtain this thing called health and wellness. This book will probably contradict everything you've been told and even things you have told others about being selfish. It's going to broaden your perspective on what's needed to obtain health from a mental, spiritual, and holistic standpoint. I will explain the science behind being Self*ish* and provide insights to help you live your best life as you achieve your health goals by becoming **Selfish.** Go ahead and get Self*ish*!

CHAPTER 2

Expressions of Spirituality

Expressions of spirituality were woven into my upbringing. When I was a child, spirituality was an integral part of my family's daily life. When I visited my paternal grandmother at her home, she would ask me to pray. She asked me to recite scriptures. We would sit together as I read and prayed for her. What a powerful way to discover the bonding power of prayer and scripture. Maybe I held a special place in my grandmother's heart as the youngest, or perhaps she illuminated my way, for her affection and care set me on a lifelong journey that I hold dear, preserving those precious early memories. I value those early memories. They predisposed me to grow spiritually. I learned that prayer is how we communicate with God and that there was no prayer that was too small or too big. While I grasped the concept of prayer, meditation, and other forms of spirituality were unfamiliar territory for me. One day, I stumbled upon my mother seated in a corner with her eyes closed. It was customary for my parents to pray, but this was different—eyes closed, complete stillness, and no words. I began to occupy myself with my Tonka truck, but a wave of fear washed over me. Was she alright? My worry grew, tears welled up, and I rushed over to her. Trembling and with teary eyes, I gently shook her. "Mom," I cried. "Are you okay?" She opened her eyes and reassured me, "I'm fine, sweetheart." I let out a sigh of relief, and she chuckled. "I was just meditating. It helps me become a better mom, a better person."

Prayer, meditation, mindful breathing, and spiritual readings are all expressions of spirituality. These expressions of spirituality during my childhood sparked a curiosity within me. As I independently engaged in these practices, I began to sense a connection between the calm they provided and a broader understanding of the human experience. This fascination eventually steered me toward delving into the science of spirituality and its potential effects on health. Exploring this realm, I discovered an intricate interplay between the mind, body, and spirit that fascinated me deeply. Through extensive research, I uncovered compelling evidence linking spiritual practices to improved mental and physical well-being. This combination of personal experience and empirical knowledge laid a strong foundation for my approach to patient care. Integrating the insights gained from spirituality and its impact on health outcomes, I developed a holistic approach that recognizes the importance of addressing not only physical ailments but also the emotional and spiritual aspects of each individual. This approach, shaped by my childhood experiences and subsequent scientific exploration, is why I told Angie she needed to find peace and that the best way was for her to get spiritual. Indeed, one of the scriptures from the Bible that I committed to memory, Matthew 6:33, encapsulates this perspective: "But seek ye first the kingdom of God, and his righteousness; and all these things shall be added unto you."

The Effect of Prayer and Meditation on the Brain

When Angie questioned the benefits and significance of prayer and meditation, I shared some enlightening research that had resonated with me. Among the many studies that deepened my understanding of the transformative power of prayer and meditation, one stood out. This particular study took a group of participants, all new to meditation, and divided them into two distinct groups. The first group continued their usual daily routines and employed their regular coping mechanisms to manage stress. The second group, on the other hand, embarked on an eight-week mindfulness meditation stress reduction program.

At the conclusion of these eight weeks, the research team utilized an MRI (magnetic resonance imaging) to measure the brain volumes of each participant in both groups, focusing on five specific brain regions. The results were nothing short of remarkable for the meditation group. In this group, four regions of the brain displayed increased thickness, akin to the growth of muscles when lifting weights, symbolizing enhanced strength—but in this case, within the brain itself.

Firstly, the posterior cingulate cortex, responsible for memory, emotional processing, introspection, and self-relevance, exhibited both increased size and thickness. Similarly, there was noticeable thickening and growth in the left hippocampus, which plays a crucial role in memory and emotional regulation. The temporal parietal junction (TPJ), associated with perspective, empathy, and compassion, also displayed increased thickness. Additionally, the pons, a region in the brainstem responsible for generating regulatory neurotransmitters, showed heightened thickness and productivity.

This groundbreaking study suggested that individuals who engaged in meditation for just two months experienced remarkable cognitive enhancements. Their minds wandered less, their ability to concentrate on tasks improved significantly, and they gained a deeper understanding of their place in the world. Conversely, those who did not meditate showed no such improvements.

As they embarked on their meditation journey, the participants' capacity for learning, critical thinking, memory recall, and overall productivity soared. Furthermore, meditation nurtured a broader perspective, fostering empathy and compassion toward others and imbuing them with a sense of purpose and love that enriched their lives. As I shared this enlightening study with Angie her demeanor softened, and she seemed more open to the idea. Encouraged by her response, I continued to discuss additional benefits of spirituality and its profound impact on overall well-being.

A study conducted at the University of Pennsylvania revealed that prayer has the remarkable ability to boost the body's dopamine levels, often referred to as the "feel-good" hormone associated with happiness. Dopamine plays a key role in motivating individuals to be active, engage in social interactions, pursue work, and contribute to their communities, all thanks to its mood-enhancing effects.

In a similar vein, research conducted at the University of Montreal demonstrated that mindfulness meditation directly influences the brain's production of serotonin. Serotonin, recognized as a natural mood stabilizer, plays a crucial role in regulating sleep, appetite, and digestion, further emphasizing the positive impact of mindfulness meditation on one's emotional well-being.

Neuroscientist Andrew Newberg, M.D., a pioneering figure in the emerging field of "neurotheology," has conducted groundbreaking research by utilizing brain scans to investigate the neurological underpinnings of religious and spiritual experiences. As a professor in the Department of Integrative Medicine and Nutritional Sciences and the director of research at the Marcus Institute of Integrative Health at Thomas Jefferson University Hospital, Dr. Newberg has unveiled important insights into the effects of religious contemplation.

His work studies individuals engaged in prayer and meditation, all aimed at unraveling the essence of religious and spiritual practices and their associated attitudes. Dr. Newberg specifically defines religious contemplation as a form of thoughtful mindfulness prayer. According to his findings, dedicating just 12 minutes daily to personal reflection and prayer can yield a profound influence on the brain.

This practice fortifies a distinctive neural circuit that not only enhances social awareness and empathy but also nurtures a heightened sense of compassion, enabling individuals to love their neighbors more deeply. Moreover, this strengthened neural circuit has the added benefit of quelling negative emotions, contributing to a more balanced and harmonious emotional state.

Spirituality and Stress

In 2013, researchers at the University of California, Davis unveiled a significant connection between mindfulness and cortisol, often referred to as the "stress hormone." Cortisol is released in response to perceived or real stress and aids the body in reacting to stressful situations. Elevated cortisol levels have been associated with heightened anxiety and depression, increased blood sugar levels, high blood pressure, inflammation, suppressed immune system function, and digestive issues like ulcers.

Remarkably, individuals who practiced mindfulness for a brief period displayed a reduction in cortisol levels. Another study conducted by Rutgers University found that meditation practitioners experienced an impressive nearly 50% reduction in cortisol levels. These findings underscore the substantial impact of meditation and mindfulness on cortisol levels and the perception of stress.

In a more recent study, participants were divided into two groups: one engaged in 40 minutes of daily meditation, and another group that maintained their regular routines and coping strategies. Each participant completed a questionnaire measuring their anxiety and stress levels, and they underwent functional magnetic resonance imaging (fMRI) to establish baseline brain activity. Three months later, the groups were retested.

The meditators reported significantly lower levels of perceived stress and anxiety compared to the non-meditators. The fMRI scans revealed changes in brain connectivity that explained this reduced anxiety and stress. The tests indicated a reconfiguration of neural connections, particularly in areas such as the precuneus, the left parietal lobe, and the insula, all of which play pivotal roles in regulating emotions and inner states. These changes were not observed in the control group, suggesting that individuals who took up meditation not only felt less stressed but also experienced neural changes that supported their perception of reduced stress. This clinical evidence underscores the impact of spirituality on stress levels.

According to a Harvard report, regular meditation practice leads to a reduction in gray matter concentration in the amygdala, the region associated with fear and stress. The amygdala plays a key role in memory recall, and when we encounter situations reminiscent of past stressors, it triggers the stress response. Those who practiced meditation regularly experienced a reduction in the size of the brain area linked to negative emotions, thus lowering stress levels typically triggered by the amygdala.

Let's delve deeper into the subject of whether spirituality, meditation, prayer, and deep breathing can effectively reduce perceived stress and improve medical conditions. This debate persists despite the existing research and anecdotal evidence that suggests these practices play a pivotal role in promoting well-being and reversing the patterns of disease. To provide further insight, the Agency for Healthcare Research and Quality conducted a study employing randomized controlled trials.

In randomized trials, subjects are divided into two groups to allow for a comparison between their outcomes after engaging in specific activities. In this instance, one group participated in mindful meditation programs while the other did not. The group that practiced meditation demonstrated modest improvements in distress levels and a positive shift in their perspective or attitude toward life, often referred to as their "negative effect."

In another study, a cardiology clinic conducted a randomized study involving 60 patients, dividing them into two groups. One group underwent an eight-week mindfulness-based stress reduction therapy, while the other group continued with their regular routines. Those who partook in mindfulness-based stress reduction reported significantly lower perceived stress levels and reduced anger compared to those in the control group.

Now, you might be wondering why addressing stress is so crucial. The reason is that stress-related ailments or challenges account for a staggering 70-90% of all physician visits. It's a remarkable statistic that underscores the necessity of addressing our stress levels if we aspire to lead healthier lives. Dealing with stress is not just an option; it is a fundamental component of overall well-being.

Stress Management, Meditation, and the Heart

A 1983 study involving 46 patients suffering from ischemic heart disease, characterized by inadequate blood flow to the heart muscle, demonstrated the remarkable benefits of a comprehensive lifestyle intervention. This approach combined stress management techniques like meditation, stretching, and relaxation with a plant-based diet. After just 24 days, participants in the lifestyle intervention group experienced impressive results, including a 44% increase in exercise duration, a 55% improvement in total work, and enhanced exercise ejection fraction, a measure of the heart's pumping strength. In contrast, there were no substantial changes observed in the control group.

Similarly, a study published in *The Journal of Nuclear Cardiology* investigated the impact of meditation, prayer, and spirituality on patients with coronary heart disease, employing PET scan imaging to assess cardiac blood flow. The findings demonstrated that individuals who integrated meditation into their heart rehabilitation routines continued to experience a more than 20% increase in cardiac blood flow compared to those who did not. While it's challenging to establish direct cause and effect, the growing body of research suggests a significant relationship between spirituality, stress, and heart disease.

Spirituality and our Arteries

Can spirituality influence the health of our arteries? Let's explore a study involving carotid intima-media thickness, where we examine the carotid arteries responsible for supplying blood to the brain. In this study, medical professionals employ ultrasound to measure the thickness of the inner layers of the carotid arteries, known as the intima and the media. This serves as a proxy indicator to assess whether individuals have atherosclerosis, a condition characterized by vascular disease, or the narrowing of blood vessels.

The research focused on 138 patients with high blood pressure, randomly assigning them to two groups: one engaging in meditation practices and the other receiving health education only. The participants were followed for seven months, although 57% dropped out, leaving 43% who completed the study. The findings revealed that those in the meditation group exhibited a regression in the buildup of arterial plaque, signifying a reduction in plaque accumulation.

Spirituality and the Effect on the Endothelium

You may remember that the endothelium is the inner lining of blood vessels responsible for preventing things from sticking or clotting to their walls. It can either promote dilation, the widening of vessels, or constriction, their narrowing. An intriguing question emerged concerning the potential influence of mindfulness-based meditation, spirituality, prayer, and deep breathing on the endothelium.

To investigate this, a prospective study, which examines future outcomes rather than past events, involved 34 female patients diagnosed with chest discomfort. After engaging in an eight-week program focused on mindfulness-based stress reduction, there were significant reductions in stress parameters and a noteworthy improvement in flow-mediated dilatation. These findings provide evidence of a link between our perception of stress, our connection to spirituality, and the impact on our blood vessels, potentially influencing outcomes such as Broken Heart Syndrome.

Breathing and Stress Reduction

I remember a session of deep muscle tissue therapy when my therapist mentioned I needed to work on my breathing. Initially surprised, I thought, *I know how to breathe!* However, my therapist explained that I wasn't taking deep breaths using my diaphragm and highlighted the intricate connection between breathing patterns and stress. This prompted me to look into the research, uncovering that stress can lead individuals to hold their breath momentarily and that chronic stress can disrupt normal breathing, causing shallow or rapid breaths even in non-stressful situations. My massage therapist recommended trying focused breathing.

Focused breathing offers a practical approach to reducing stress, serving as an alternative to prayer and meditation. The term "spirit" in spirituality originates from the Latin word "spiritus," meaning breath, highlighting the natural connection between focused breathing and spirituality. In this practice, individuals deliberately engage in slow, deep breaths—inhaling through the nose and exhaling through the mouth. Attention is directed toward the sensory experience of breathing, encompassing the flow of air in and out, the rhythmic expansion and contraction of the chest and abdomen, or the gentle sensation of breath passing over the nostrils or lips. Focused breathing cultivates a heightened awareness of thoughts and emotions, fostering inner peace and tranquility. Research suggests that, much like prayer and meditation, breathing techniques can effectively alleviate symptoms associated with stress-related disorders, including anxiety, general stress, depression, and post-traumatic stress disorder.

Breathing techniques exert influence on both physiological factors within the body and psychological factors in the brain and our thoughts. This explains why people often take a deep breath before confronting a stressful event, such as giving a presentation or facing a test. A recent study demonstrates that students who employ breathing techniques in response to stress exhibit greater activation in the prefrontal cortex, the brain region responsible for processing thoughts. Participants using these techniques displayed improved control of amygdala activity and reduced cortisol levels, the stress hormone. Focusing on your breath not only enhances your willpower but also diminishes your stress response.

One effective way to initiate the breathing response is through the physiologic sigh—a pattern involving a long inhale followed by a shorter one, followed by a slow exhale through the mouth. Research underscores the significance of physiologic sighs in regulating the body's response to stress. Stress activates the sympathetic nervous system (the fight or flight response), which can lead to hyperventilation and decreased carbon dioxide levels in the blood, resulting in anxiety and panic. Physiologic sighs help counteract this by increasing carbon dioxide levels, which calms the body and reduces stress and anxiety. Studies further reveal that slow, deep breaths akin to physiologic sighs can reduce other physiological markers of stress, including heart rate and blood pressure.

Sel*fish* Tip

Do box breathing when you are stressed. Box breathing, also known as square breathing or four-square breathing, is a relaxation technique that involves taking slow, deep breaths in a pattern of four equal parts. The technique is commonly used to reduce stress and anxiety and to promote calmness. Start by exhaling completely and then inhaling through your nose for a count of four. Hold your breath for a count of four. Exhale slowly through your mouth for a count of four. Hold your breath again for a count of four. Repeat the pattern for a few minutes or as long as you need to feel calm and relaxed.

Science-based evidence tells us that adopting these strategies will lower our stress response.

Spirituality and Willpower

Our willpower is closely connected to our keystone habits. Charles Duhigg's book *The Power of Habit* underscores how these foundational habits significantly impact our work, diet, leisure, lifestyle, spending patterns, and communication. By consistently practicing these habits over time, they can gradually reshape different aspects of our lives. Additionally, practices such as meditation and prayer, which fall under the umbrella of spirituality, contribute to enhancing our willpower and facilitating personal transformation.

An example of this can be seen in a study that examined 20 Alcoholics Anonymous members who had successfully resisted the urge to drink for a week. Using MRI scans, they were shown alcohol-related advertisements and scenes of people drinking while their responses were measured. These visuals were presented after reading neutral news and after reciting an Alcoholics Anonymous prayer that promotes abstinence. Following exposure to the images, all participants reported some desire to drink, yet this craving lessened after reciting the AA prayer. The MRI findings are particularly intriguing, revealing changes in the brain's prefrontal cortex, a region responsible for managing stress, emotions, and our comprehension of feelings. This study highlights not only the impact of prayer on reducing cravings in the context of addiction recovery but also the broader potential of prayer as a tool for managing and mitigating stress. Engaging in spiritual or mindfulness practices like prayer can help individuals cultivate inner calm, emotional balance, and coping strategies to better handle the stressors of daily life.

Another study investigating keystone habits and willpower conducted a comprehensive review of 21 separate studies involving over 300 participants. The outcomes revealed consistent changes in brain regions among individuals who practiced meditation. These alterations affected regions pivotal to meta-awareness, body awareness, and self- and emotional regulation. Moreover, structural changes were identified in various brain components of those who meditated, such as the cerebral cortex, subcortical gray and white matter, brain stem, and cerebellum. This suggests the intriguing possibility that willpower can be bolstered similarly to building a muscle through practices like meditation and prayer. Strengthening willpower enables individuals to manage their emotions and attain their goals effectively.

The Spirituality of "Getting Self*ish*"

You may wonder how you can incorporate getting Self*ish* into your busy life—I did, too. On my plate were a busy clinical practice, a wife, two children, administrative work, and a passion for the community. Despite my love for them all, I too have felt stressed and overwhelmed. As I shared with Angie the power of the "S" in spiritual, I too felt motivated to start as well.

It has been a journey where I've learned that the secret sauce to building a new habit or practice of being spiritual is to understand it is not about perfection. It's about being intentional. Start out by identifying the easiest thing to accomplish, something you know that you will and can do. What is the smallest task you can be successful at? James Clear, in his book *Atomic Habits*, talks about how small changes transform our habits and deliver amazing results. Starting or changing small habits are a part of the equation, but developing SMART goals is equally important. SMART goals are goals that are specific, measurable, achievable, relevant, and have a time limit.

Your belief system will determine whether you use meditation, prayer, or simply breathing techniques. A 2005 study in the *Journal of Behavioral Medicine* that compared secular and spiritual forms of meditation found spiritual meditation to be more calming than secular meditation. Secular meditation means focusing on your breath or focusing on a non-spiritual word such as "relax." In spiritual meditation, you focus on God or a spiritual word or phrase. Participants were divided into two groups. One group was taught to meditate using words of self-affirmation, such as "I am love," while others were taught to meditate using words describing a higher power, such as "God is love." Each group meditated 20 minutes a day for four weeks. Researchers found that the group that practiced spiritual meditation showed greater decreases in anxiety and stress. Their moods were more positive in those who were dependent on God. They also tolerated discomfort almost twice as long when asked to put their hands in ice water. The choice is yours whether you choose meditation, prayer, or deep breathing, but once you decide on how you will get spiritual, you will need to answer these questions to keep yourself accountable: How will you measure your goal? How will you track it and stay committed to your practice on a regular basis? One option is to use an app. There are apps for meditation, breathing, and prayer, complete with timers to encourage consistent use. You may want to form or join a like-minded group for added support. If you're not using an app, journaling about your efforts can be effective. Make sure when you set your goals that they are attainable. But remember, set attainable goals and a consistent process. If you're new to meditation, prayer, or focused breathing, aiming for an hour daily might be unrealistic. Start small, then gradually build. Firmly establishing the process is paramount. For instance, you might consider setting a goal to engage in five minutes of meditation/prayer or focused breathing every day for a month. However, it's not solely about dedicating time; it involves embracing the entire process. Ensure a firm commitment not only to the duration but also to the specifics of when, where, and how you will engage in your chosen practice, whether it's prayer, meditation, or focused breathing. The path may be gradual, but it's a steadfast way to integrate the spirituality of Self*ish* into your busy life. Find more information to guide your action plan at www.DrBatiste.com.

CHAPTER 3

Exercise

Some of my earliest memories of my dad are from the times he played with me. In today's vernacular, it would be called exercise. My dad was fiercely competitive and wouldn't let me win just because I was his son. It didn't matter if we were playing Uno, ping pong, football, or basketball, he wasn't going to let me win until I could really beat him. This is what fuels my competitive fire to this day. I cherish those moments I had with my dad, being active. I don't know how he knew precisely when to take me out for a game of one-on-one basketball, but as I look back, we typically went out when I was feeling a bit grumpy or sad. After a little time in the sun and running around, my grumpy, sullen teenage mode would improve—especially when I started to beat him. Fast forward some 30 years, and I've found myself mimicking my dad. It was not a conscious reflex, I just acted.

I have a vivid memory of a day from when my daughter Brooke was in her early teenage years. As many parents, aunts, or uncles can relate, those early teen years often come with a challenging attitude. It's a phase marked by pervasive mood swings, and if they're not talking back, they tend to withdraw into silence.

On this particular day, I decided to take action and suggested that Brooke and I go for a walk. Of course she said no, but with a little parental persuasion, she agreed. She seemed closed off and distant; however, as we started our walk in the sun among the trees, a transformation began. Her initial frown gradually softened, and the tension in her fists and folded arms eased. With time, she even started to laugh at my dad jokes and began sharing her thoughts and feelings.

By the end of our walk, the shift in Brooke's mood was remarkable. She told me I was right and that she felt better after going on the walk. This experience underscored the power of exercise.

I told Angie about that walk with my daughter as we sat in my office. I added, "Exercise is one of the most powerful therapies I can prescribe. It can transform your mood, improve your health, and drain away your fatigue as it reinvigorates you. Will you consider exercising as part of your treatment?" Talk about deja vu. I thought I was talking to my 13-year-old teenage daughter. If looks could kill. She was resistant and skeptical. Angie looked at me and confided, "I'm self-conscious about my weight, and the thought of it brings back memories of when my ex-husband and I used to walk together, which makes me feel worse. To be honest, my schedule is packed. I don't have the energy, and I'm not sure exercise can truly make a difference." Frustration colored her tone, and her eyes welled up with tears as she concluded, "I'm not like your teenage daughter, and I'm just not convinced that this approach is effective."

"Angie," I replied, "Remember there is power in being selfish. One of the key pillars of Self*ish* is exercise. Exercise is a core ingredient in curing stress and Broken Heart Syndrome. If you trust me, then trust the process. Exercise is therapeutic."

Exercise as a Foundational Practice

Angie was a bit curious at this point. "Why is exercise a

foundational practice?" she asked.

I replied, "Because it's a keystone habit. Have you ever read the book The Power of Habit by Charles Duhigg?"

She looked at me inquisitively. "No."

I went on. In the book, Duhigg explains that keystone habits change more than just our behavior. They change how we see ourselves. When researchers examine how individuals alter their habitual behaviors, it's the keystone habits that trigger a ripple effect, leading to changes in other life patterns.

Exercise is indeed this golden keystone habit. Exercise is a springboard or platform on which other healthy habits are built on. Exercise as a keystone habit can be understood from Colcombe et al.'s study in 2006 on the anterior midcingulate cortex (aMCC). The anterior midcingulate cortex (aMCC) is a brain region associated with motivation, persistence, and decision-making. Research suggests that individuals with strong willpower and persistence often exhibit greater activity in the aMCC. This brain region may be crucial in driving behavior and sustaining efforts towards long-term goals, such as maintaining a regular exercise routine or eating healthfully. Colcombe et al. conducted a study involving older adults who participated in aerobic exercise, calisthenics, and stretching activities. They found that individuals who engaged in moderate-intensity aerobic exercise experienced maintenance or even an increase in their anterior midcingulate cortex size. This suggests that regular aerobic exercise may positively impact the structure and function of the aMCC. The findings from Colcombe et al.'s study provides insight into how exercise can influence brain health, specifically in regions associated with motivation and persistence. By engaging in regular exercise, individuals may not only improve their physical fitness but also enhance their cognitive function and mental resilience. This, in turn, can contribute to developing a keystone habit where the positive effects of exercise extend beyond physical health to influence various aspects of daily life. According to research, regular exercise serves as a trigger for people to eat healthier, to have more patience, to be less stressed, to consume less alcohol, to smoke less, and even to become more productive at work. Exercise contributes to a better mood and improves sleep quality. When you build a habit of daily exercise, you not only improve your health and fitness, but you also create a new self-image. This impression of who you are and who you want to be is that of a person who exercises regularly. You want the self-image of a healthy person. By starting with action that encourages the self-image, we subconsciously encourage ourselves to reinforce that new self-image." Angie nodded her head as if she was considering what I said.

Exercise and Mood

Angie's eyes were glued on me as I spoke and she finally blurted out, "Can exercise really change your mood? Can it make you happy?" What happens to your brain when you exercise?

I knew I had her. I responded, "Interesting you should ask. There's a study involving numerous countries around the world that indicates that as little as 10 minutes of physical activity per week can increase your level of happiness."

When you start to exercise, within just 5 minutes of moving your body, your brain receives an instant boost. During this time, as your heart rate and breathing gradually increase, more oxygen and nutrients are carried to your brain, promoting the growth of new neurons.

Around 20 to 30 minutes into your workout, feel-good hormones called endorphins and endocannabinoids are released. These chemicals help improve mood, stress response, memory, and more, contributing to the overall feel-good effect of exercise.

After about 60 minutes, the production of an important brain chemical called brain-derived neurotrophic factor (BDNF) increases, especially with high-intensity interval training (HIIT). BDNF helps our brains work correctly, enhancing mood, learning, and memory. It's like a substance that improves traffic and communication within the brain while also encouraging brain growth. Even a single HIIT workout can temporarily boost focus and concentration.

Between 2 to 4 hours post-exercise, another wave of brain chemicals is released, including serotonin, dopamine, and norepinephrine. These neurotransmitters play a crucial role in delivering messages between neurons.

Over the course of 12 weeks or more, regular aerobic or HIIT sessions can lead to sustained increase in BDNF production. This can positively impact brain size, particularly in areas associated with memory.

After 3 or more months of consistent exercise, your brain and body become healthier. Exercise increases insulin-like growth factor 1 (IGF-1), which helps stabilize blood sugar levels and improve insulin sensitivity. This can have a positive impact on cognitive health since poor metabolic health is linked to cognitive decline. Essentially, the way your body processes sugar is connected to brain health, highlighting the importance of exercise for both physical and cognitive well-being.

Remember this important point: We don't find time to exercise; we make time to exercise! Physical activity improves mental health, reduces diabetes, and improves heart disease and cancer. Despite that, less than half of Americans exercise as much as they should. I want to change that.

Despite its benefits, exercise is a stressor on the body, but it's almost like going to training camp to prepare for a football or basketball game. When you train your body to manage stress levels, it makes your body more resilient. The body is used to dealing with stress, because stress provides the signal for the body to secrete hormones so it can take action. The body prepares us for fighting or fleeing. That's the stress hormone cascade. I mentioned previously the research that shows that the stress response spikes initially but then abates. People then experience lower levels of stress hormones like cortisol and epinephrine after bouts of physical activity.

Perceived stress is a person's feelings and thoughts about the level of stress they are experiencing currently or over a period of time. Angie asked, "Can exercise really reduce the stress I'm experiencing in life?" I wanted to drive this point home, so I shared several pertinent studies.

There was a study published in Biological Research for Nursing that studied whether or not exercise had an impact on perceived stress. They also looked at markers of inflammation, the things that can lead to disease that are triggered by stress. The researchers took two groups; one group walked 30 minutes a day for 10 weeks and the other group kept their sedentary routine. The exercise group reported significant improvements in their stress, their mood, and their quality of life compared to the sedentary group. Here's the most significant part of the study as it relates to health: The exercise group demonstrated a decrease in markers of inflammation that have been shown to be associated with heart disease. This was a pivotal study that was foundational for subsequent studies.

Another study looked at individuals who exercise two or three times per week. They certainly were not marathon runners or super athletes. What they found was that the individuals who exercised the most had less depression, anger, cynicism, and stress compared to those who exercised less or not at all.

Another study brought to light that sedentary individuals were three times more likely to have perceived stress than those who were active and engaged. People who work, which is most of us, and participate in a moderate amount of physical activity have half the rate of perceived stress as those who are inactive. These studies provide authoritative evidence of the effectiveness of exercise. One study revealed that students who participated in a research-designed aerobic training program reduced their stress, anxiety, and depression.

During medical school, the amount of information we had to learn was overwhelming. The ever-present need to study reams of information, the lack of sleep, and the pressure to do well in school was crushing. We had no time for ourselves, and our relationships were strained. I felt stretched in every direction. It was the exercise that saw me through. Exercise brought me through my times of challenge as a youth, and those lessons surrounding the power of exercise my dad taught me served me well during the demanding days of medical school. In short, exercise is powerful medicine, and it's free!

Exercise and a Broken Heart

Angie sat in the office, her heart racing with anxiety as I suggested she start exercising. The mere thought of it filled her with fear, especially given her diagnosis of heart failure. She was afraid to move, scared that any exertion would worsen her condition and lead to a catastrophic event.

I shared that the medical community has come a long way in understanding heart disease and exercise. I acknowledged her concerns and told her how long-ago physicians (in the 18th Century) treated heart attacks with bed rest for at least a month to aid in healing. This approach persisted into the mid-20th century, with patients often confined to bed for over six weeks after heart attacks, followed by restricted physical activity for up to a year. By the late 20th century, the understanding of the role of physical activity in heart attack recovery evolved, moving away from strict bed rest towards more active rehabilitation strategies.

I further explained to her that when a person exercises, their cardiovascular system goes into action to meet the increased demand for oxygen and nutrients in their body's tissues. The heart starts beating faster, pumping more oxygen-rich blood to the muscles, and working hard. This increased heart rate helps deliver oxygen and nutrients to the muscles more efficiently. With each heartbeat, the heart pumps more blood, known as stroke volume. This means that with each beat, more blood is sent out to the body's tissues, helping to meet the increased demand for oxygen and nutrients during exercise. The blood vessels dilate during exercise allowing more blood to flow through them. This helps deliver oxygen and nutrients to the muscles and removes waste products more efficiently. These changes in the cardiovascular system during exercise help ensure that the body's tissues receive enough oxygen and nutrients to support physical activity.

Exercise and Endothelial Function

I reminded Angie how the endothelium is a portal to health. I told her how exercise plays a crucial role in improving the function of the endothelium, which is essential for heart health. Vascular endothelial dysfunction, a key factor in conditions like atherosclerosis, where arteries narrow due to plaque buildup, can be countered through exercise. By increasing the production of nitric oxide (NO) in blood vessel linings, exercise enhances their ability to dilate, promoting smoother blood flow. Regular aerobic activities such as running or biking can increase artery widening by 2% to 4%. Athletes who maintain consistent activity typically have larger arteries than less active individuals. Even starting exercise later in life, with as little as 8 weeks of aerobic activity, can enhance artery flexibility and thickness, reducing blockage risks. Moreover, aerobic exercise can decrease artery stiffness, a risk factor for heart disease.

Research also indicates positive effects of resistance training, like weightlifting, on blood vessel function, bone loss prevention, and muscle mass preservation. Studies show that resistance training improves flow-mediated dilation (FMD), indicating better blood vessel performance, across various health conditions. Continuous aerobic exercises, particularly of moderate to vigorous intensity like running or biking, are effective in enhancing blood vessel function. Longer exercise durations, older age, higher BMI, and poorer initial blood vessel function correlate with more significant improvements post-exercise. Overall, regular aerobic exercise benefits blood vessel health, with additional benefits from resistance training, irrespective of health conditions.

Exercise & Ischemic Heart Disease

The question surrounding what physical activities a patient can perform after a heart attack is still one of the most common questions I receive when caring for patients. To be honest, I love this question because it provides me an opportunity to share some of the rich history surrounding exercise and heart disease. The events surrounding President Eisenhower are seminal moments in the history and treatment of heart disease.

In 1955, President Dwight D. Eisenhower had a heart attack while visiting his mother-in-law. This event had a significant impact on the country, especially on the financial markets. The news caused panic on Wall Street, leading to a significant drop in stock prices. Dr. Paul Dudley White, a prominent cardiologist, played a key role in Eisenhower's care. He believed in getting patients up and moving soon after a heart attack, which was different from the usual advice of prolonged bed rest. Despite criticism, Dr. White's approach proved groundbreaking and changed how heart attacks are treated. Nowadays, patients with uncomplicated heart attacks spend only a short time in the hospital, thanks to Dr. White's pioneering methods.

Reflecting, it appears the events surrounding President Eisenhower were a springboard to many of the technological advances in treating heart disease, but it was also a launchpad to the power of exercise. The research surrounding the benefits of exercise in patients with coronary artery disease has exploded since the 1950s. Regular exercise offers significant advantages for individuals with coronary artery disease (CAD). Research indicates that exercise-based rehabilitation can notably lower the likelihood of death from CAD up to 63%. For instance, the STABILITY study, involving more than 15,000 CAD patients, revealed that those who engaged in more physical activity experienced fewer heart-related issues over a span of three years. Even incorporating just two hours of brisk walking per week can yield positive effects. Exercise is particularly beneficial for individuals at elevated risk of heart problems, such as older adults, smokers, or those with conditions like high cholesterol or diabetes.

The type of exercise also plays a crucial role. More intense workouts that induce a feeling of breathlessness tend to be the most effective. For individuals with significant blockages in their coronary arteries, regular exercise can enhance their capacity to engage in physical activity without discomfort, diminish the necessity for hospital visits, and decrease the likelihood of requiring additional surgeries.

Exercise operates by reducing the buildup of plaque in the arteries, thereby enhancing their stability and enhancing blood flow. Additionally, it aids in the improvement of the functionality of the small blood vessels surrounding the heart. A study found that just four weeks of exercise led to improvements in these small blood vessels among CAD patients.

Overall, these findings underscore the importance of regular and challenging exercise in enhancing heart health and reducing the risk of heart issues in individuals with CAD. Additionally, exercise capacity emerged as a superior predictor of death at both two and five years compared to the squeezing capacity or left ventricular ejection fraction (LVEF) in patients sustaining a major heart attack called ST-elevation myocardial infarction (STEMI) who underwent treatment with stents.

Exercise and Heart Failure

"I'm still scared," Angie admitted. The thought of exercising brought up emotional memories, but beyond that, she feared that her heart might suffer if she committed to physical activity. Angie knew she needed to start her journey in using exercise as a therapy, but she was frozen in fear. I suggested cardiac rehabilitation (CR). CR is a comprehensive program that includes exercise training, health education, cardiovascular risk management, and psychological support tailored to the individual needs of patients with heart disease.

I assured Angie that CR could be a beneficial starting point, especially considering her history of Broken Heart Syndrome. Broken Heart Syndrome occurs when the nervous system becomes too active, leading to harmful chemical surges that can damage the heart. Aerobic exercises, like walking or biking, which are a key component of CR, can help reduce these harmful chemicals and lower blood pressure. Research shows that even minor improvements in exercise capacity can decrease the risk of death. Therefore, structured exercise programs in CR can help Broken Heart Syndrome patients exercise better and regulate these harmful chemical responses.

Acknowledging Angie's feelings of stress and depression, I reminded her that she wasn't alone. People with Broken Heart Syndrome often experience similar emotions and symptoms akin to those who have had a heart attack. CR has been proven to improve depression and stress levels, providing valuable support for individuals like Angie. Recent studies have shown significant improvements in functional exercise capacity and exercise time for heart failure patients participating in phase II CR programs.

Additionally, exercise has been found to positively affect the health of people with stable heart failure (HF). Moderate-intensity continuous training (MICT) combined with resistance training has shown efficacy. Large-scale trials such as the HF-ACTION trial have demonstrated that exercise training can slightly reduce the risk of death or hospitalization in HF patients. Short-term rehabilitation, as seen in studies like REHAB-HF, can also enhance physical performance in elderly HF patients after a period of worsening symptoms. High-intensity interval training (HIIT) has emerged as another beneficial form of exercise for people with stable HF with reduced ejection fraction (HFrEF). Studies like SMARTEX-HF have shown that HIIT can improve heart function and aerobic capacity, similar to MICT. Overall, both MICT and HIIT can be valuable tools for improving exercise capacity and overall health in people with stable HFrEF.

Exercise and Chronic Disease

Feeling comfortable about her heart being able to tolerate exercise, Angie asked, "What about my Diabetes and Weight? Will exercise help them as well?"   Angie, I understand your concern about whether exercise can help your chronic disease. Let's discuss how exercise can benefit different health conditions.

First, let's discuss diabetes. Diabetes is like being dressed up to go to a party with a date escorting you, but when you get there, the venue is filled. Blood sugar (you dressed up for a party) circulates in the bloodstream, and insulin is the key (or escort) to get blood sugar into cells. One hypothesis is that the cells are filled with fat or intramyocellular lipid , which prevents entry, causing the sugar to remain in the vessels, which can be harmful to your body, especially your heart. But exercise is like a superhero for people with diabetes! It helps lower your blood sugar levels and keeps your heart healthy. Studies have shown that exercise, both aerobic and resistance training, can significantly lower hemoglobin A1c levels (a measure of the percent of red blood cells that are crystallized from circulating blood sugar) in patients with type 2 diabetes mellitus (T2DM). This improvement in glycemic control is crucial because it can help reduce the risk of cardiovascular events and mortality associated with T2DM. Additionally, even light walking after a meal, in as little as two to five-minute increments, has been found to have a significant impact on moderating blood sugar levels.

Next, let's talk about hypertension, which is like watering your lawn with a fireman's hose on full blast vs a garden hose. Just like the pressure from the fireman's hose can cause damage to the top layer of the grass, high blood pressure can strain your heart and arteries. Exercise acts like a valve, releasing some of that pressure and keeping your heart and arteries healthy. Both aerobic and resistance exercise training have been shown to decrease blood pressure by about 5 to 7 mm Hg. While these reductions might seem small, they are essential for health and are similar to the effects of certain blood pressure medications. Lowering systolic BP by just 5 mm Hg has been shown to decrease the risk of heart problems by 10% in people with normal and high BP.

High cholesterol is like having too much grease in your pipes, which can clog them up and cause problems. Exercise acts like a scrub brush, cleaning out those pipes and keeping your arteries clear and your heart healthy. Studies show that exercise can increase high-density lipoprotein (HDL) cholesterol by 2 to 5 mg/dL, lower low-density lipoprotein (LDL) cholesterol by 3 to 10 mg/dL, and decrease fasting triglycerides by 5 to 25 mg/dL. While these changes may seem small compared to cholesterol-lowering medications like statins, both statins and exercise can independently lower the risk of death in people with high cholesterol. Most of the benefits from exercise are likely due to improved fitness levels rather than changes in blood fats, but exercise might also directly help protect arteries from clogging in people with high cholesterol.

Now, let's discuss weight loss. It's like shedding some extra baggage that's been weighing you down, both physically and mentally. Exercise is like a magic wand that helps melt away those pounds and inches, leaving you feeling lighter and more energetic. While long-term aerobic exercise may not cause significant drops in body weight, it can help reduce dangerous types of fat around the organs, which are closely linked to higher risks of heart disease and type 2 diabetes.

Overall, exercise plays a crucial role in managing chronic diseases like diabetes, hypertension, high cholesterol, and weight loss. It's a powerful pillar in Self*ish* that can improve your heart health and overall well-being.

A Journey of a Thousand Miles

In embarking on your journey towards a healthier lifestyle through exercise, remember the wisdom of the proverb: "A journey of a thousand miles begins with the first step." In this journey, adopting a SMART approach is essential. SMART stands for Specific, Measurable, Achievable, Relevant, and Time-bound, and it's a powerful framework for setting and achieving goals. Begin by setting specific and realistic goals, focusing on what you want to achieve with your exercise routine. Ensure that your goals are measurable, allowing you to track your progress over time, whether it's the number of minutes you exercise or the distance you cover. Start with small, achievable goals, like committing to just 5 minutes of exercise each day instead of aiming for a daunting 30-minute session. By starting small, you build momentum and confidence, setting yourself up for success. Remember to keep your goals relevant to your overall health and wellness objectives. Finally, set a timeframe for reaching each goal, creating a sense of urgency and accountability. Embrace the process of planning and refining your approach to exercise, recognizing that progress is made one step at a time. So, challenge yourself to adopt a SMART approach to exercise, starting with small, achievable goals and focusing on the process as much as the outcome. Always keep in mind that your journey to improved fitness begins with that very first step. For additional tips on integrating exercise into your routine to alleviate stress and foster emotional healing, connect with our community at www.DrBatiste.com.

CHAPTER 4

Love

"I don't believe in love anymore," Angie remarked. Angie's cynical perspective caught me off guard. Her words hit me hard, and I struggled to respond. As a heart doctor, I knew that her beliefs could harm her well-being. Without thinking, I felt compelled to intervene and said, "Angie, love is not just a noun that identifies a fleeting feeling. If you believe that, then you're right—love can disappear like a day-old Snapchat message. But love is more than that. Love is a verb. It's an expression, an act, a current, and a way of being. Love is forgiveness. It's gratitude, and it requires hard work to keep it alive. It's not always pretty, and it often involves pushing through pain, but that's what makes it powerful. You know this because you've experienced love before, both giving and receiving. So don't give up on love just yet."

Angie maintained her skepticism, and her eyes remained fixed on me as she persisted in her assertion that love did not exist. Realizing that I needed to change my approach, I decided to abandon my "doctor's coat" and instead put on my "lawyer gear" to make my case. Through my research, I discovered that there is a science behind romantic love known as eros—the very type of love that Angie was talking about. However, I also recognized that Angie's understanding of love was limited and narrow, and so I felt compelled to broaden her perspective by delving deeper into the topic of love.

Let us explore the subject of love more thoroughly. In my research, I started by exploring the work of Dr. Helen Fisher, a renowned biological anthropologist with a Ph.D., whose extensive publications explore the neurochemistry of romantic love and attachment. Dr. Fisher, along with her research team at Rutgers University, categorized love into three distinct types: lust, attraction, and attachment, with lust and attraction belonging to the eros or romantic love category, often characterized by its tendency to diminish over time in a relationship, while the third type, attachment, plays a distinct role in lasting relationships.

Each category of love is characterized by a unique set of messengers, or hormones, that the body employs to communicate with other organs and elicit a response. Similar to how Snapchat automatically deletes messages after 24 hours, these hormones disappear once they have fulfilled their messaging role. Lust, a phase driven by hormones, creates a longing for intimacy. Testosterone and estrogen are the hormones that drive lust. Testosterone is well-known for its role in sexual desire, with higher levels of this hormone being linked to increased sexual desire and activity in both men and women. Estrogen also plays a role in sexual desire, with higher levels of this hormone being associated with greater sexual desire and activity in women, particularly during the ovulatory phase of the menstrual cycle. Recent research has suggested that estrogen may influence the brain's reward system, which is responsible for feelings of pleasure and motivation.

Attraction is fueled by the hormones dopamine, norepinephrine, and serotonin. Dopamine is responsible for the reward pathway, or the feel-good neurotransmitter that underlies attraction. During the attraction phase, there is an increased blood flow to the brain's pleasure center, which is why we become fixated on pleasure-seeking. When we are attracted to someone, whether it's that charming guy or that charismatic girl, we experience a pleasurable feeling that makes us happy. This feeling is something we crave and repeatedly seek, as it is caused by the release of dopamine when we engage in activities that make us feel good.

Another hormone that comes into play during the attraction phase is norepinephrine. Norepinephrine causes us to feel giddy and energetic, creating that sensation of the heart skipping a beat. It is responsible for our preoccupation with the person we are attracted to, and once we have experienced its intoxicating effects, we yearn to feel it again.

Serotonin is the mood and social hormone. Low levels of serotonin have been linked to feelings of longing or infatuation for someone. In the early stages of attraction, when a person is infatuated with someone, they may experience an increase in dopamine and a decrease in serotonin levels. This decrease in serotonin levels has been linked to obsessive thoughts and behaviors toward the object of attraction.

The evolution of imaging technology like functional magnetic resonance imaging (fMRI) has given behavioral scientists like Dr. Fisher a new playground to test their hypotheses. fMRI is a non-invasive imaging technique that uses a strong magnetic field and radio waves to detect changes in blood flow and oxygenation in the brain. It is used to study brain function by measuring the activity of neurons in response to different stimuli or tasks. Studies involving fMRIs show that the reward centers of the brain activate when people see a photo of someone that they are intensely attracted to compared to when shown someone they feel neutral toward. This attraction leads to a reduction in serotonin, which leads scientists to speculate that this is what underlies the overpowering infatuation that characterizes the beginning stages of love.

The duration of periods of lust and attraction can vary from person to person and can be influenced by a range of factors, including individual differences, relationship dynamics, and life circumstances. In general, the initial period of intense attraction and infatuation, also known as the "honeymoon phase," typically lasts between six months and two years. After the honeymoon phase, the intensity of these feelings may start to diminish, and individuals may shift to a more stable and comfortable phase of the relationship—the attachment phase. Although Dr. Fisher hypothesized that the lust and attraction phase dissipates over time, I can say that after 25 years of marriage, my heart still skips a beat and I long for my wife when she is not nearby ☺.

The third type of love is known as attachment. This phase is often marked by an increase in the levels of the hormone oxytocin, which is associated with feelings of bonding and attachment. Attachment is the foundation of friendships, parent-infant bonding, and many other types of close relationships. The two primary hormones involved in attachment are oxytocin and vasopressin. Oxytocin, often referred to as the "cuddle hormone," is released in large amounts during sexual intercourse, breastfeeding, and childbirth, all of which serve as precursors to bonding. These hormones flood the body with an overwhelming sense of well-being and security that are conducive to forming lasting relationships. It can enhance feelings of social connection and reduce the physiological and emotional effects of stress. The attachment phase is sustainable, and losing someone with whom we are bonded can result in a loss of that sense of well-being. In the words of the Righteous Brothers: *"You lost that lovin' feelin'; Whoa, that lovin' feelin'; You lost that lovin' feelin'; Now it's gone, gone, gone, whoa-oh."*

Whoa-oh is right. When Angie said she didn't believe in love, what she meant was that she'd lost that lovin' feelin'. The death of her mother and the broken bond from the end of her marital relationship lowered her oxytocin levels and subsequently her sense of well-being.

What Does Love Really Mean?

During our conversations about Angie's perspective on love, I began to wonder if her lack of belief in love was because of our overuse of the word in everyday practice. Nowadays, we frequently use the word "love" to describe our affinity for a variety of things, such as food, TV shows, or even inanimate objects. We use the word love so frequently that anyone learning the English language might be confused by what people mean by the word love. When we look at the ancient Greeks, they, too, would be confused by our use of the word love. They had four different words to describe the diverse emotions we associate with love. They used *philia*, *eros*, *storge*, and *agape* to express different forms of love. Our contemporary use of love has diluted its significance.

Philia is the first of the Greek words for love. When we look at the word *philia*, it's easy to guess what this word means because it is the root word in Philadelphia, the city of brotherly love. *Philia* describes the type of love found in strong friendships. It refers to a love based on mutual respect, shared decisions, joint interests, and common values. It is the love of near and dear friends. The defining feature of *philia,* or friendship, is goodwill, which is less dependent on our individual qualities than other forms of love. Instead, *philia* arises from a sense of familiarity and connection with others.

Eros is the second of the Greek words for love. *Eros* differs from philia in that it is a passionate love, a burning love, the love found in romantic relationships. It is the lust and attraction phase of love we described earlier. In Greek mythology, it is said to be a form of madness brought about by one of Cupid's arrows, the arrow that reaches us as we fall deeply in love. In the Greek story of Paris, while he was visiting Sparta, he saw Helen, the wife of King Menelaus, and was instantly smitten with her. In some versions of the myth, Cupid, the Roman god of love, was responsible for this instant attraction by striking Paris with his arrow. Paris, unable to resist his love for Helen, abducted her and took her back to Troy with him. This sparked the Trojan War, as Menelaus and the Greeks fought to reclaim Helen and avenge her kidnapping.

Storge is the third word the Greeks used for love. It refers to familial love, particularly the love between parents and their children, or the love between siblings. *Storge* is typically characterized as a gentle, nurturing, and unconditional type of love. *Storge* can blend with and help underpin other types of love, such as *eros*. It is often depicted as a natural and instinctual love, arising from the biological ties and shared experiences of family members. While *storge* is generally associated with familial relationships, it can also extend to other types of relationships that share a similar bond of care and affection, such as close friendships or even relationships with pets.

Agape love is the fourth word the Greeks used for love. It is a Greek term that refers to a selfless, unconditional, and altruistic love that seeks the highest good for another person, without any expectation of receiving something in return. It is a universal love. This type of love is often associated with spiritual and religious contexts, as it is often described as the type of love that God has for humanity. The Christian faith calls it charity and identifies *agape* as the highest form of love. *Agape* love involves sacrificing one's own desires, needs, and interests to serve and care for another person, regardless of whether that person deserves it or reciprocates the same level of affection. It is a love that transcends personal biases, prejudices, and preferences and seeks to promote the well-being of others. In essence, *agape* love is a form of love that is based on empathy, compassion, and altruism, and it is focused on the well-being and happiness of the other person rather than on personal gain or pleasure. *Agape* helps build and maintain the psychological, social, and environmental fabric of society. This fabric forms a shield that sustains and enriches us. *Agape* is much more than a feeling or sentiment. *Agape* is the true definition of love in action. Our world seems to be steeped in continual crisis: the pandemic, wars, rumors of wars, and natural calamities. There's always strife, civil unrest, and increasing anger and division. Considering the state of our planet, we need more altruism, or *agape*.

The Language of Love

What is so interesting is that as I transitioned from investigating the science of love to reading about the history of love, my mind began to reflect on my own love story. I met the love of my life in college. I still remember the moment I first saw her, one Friday night in front of a place called Moran Hall on the campus of a Historically Black College and University, Oakwood College. I remember all the feelings of the new love: the dopaminergic drive to be around her like a moth to a light; the butterfly feelings from the surge of norepinephrine and the feelings of melancholy when I wasn't around her. The funny part is that this occurred before we even started to date. After I somehow convinced her to start a relationship with me, I quickly realized that some of the things I was doing to show her how much I "loved" her wasn't giving her that loving feeling. It wasn't that "men are from Mars and women are from Venus," it was because I wasn't speaking *her* love language. That's when my brother, who is 16 years my senior (yes, I love to mention that I'm the youngest of my siblings, which means I had the opportunity to learn from them), gave me a book that transformed my relationship: *The Five Love Languages* by Gary Chapman.

Gary Chapman introduced five categories in his inaugural book, *The Five Love Languages*, to describe how individuals express and receive love: Words of Affirmation, Quality Time,

Receiving Gifts, Acts of Service, and Physical Touch. According to Chapman, everyone has each of the five languages, but most people have one primary language that they use to express and receive love. Each aspect of the love language is crucial and can be prioritized based on personal preferences.

In addition to helping individuals with their relationships, I suggested to Angie that effectively using the five love languages could also aid in the healing process for those with a broken and stressed heart.

Words of Affirmation and the Heart

The power of words of affirmation has been put to the test through research. In one study, researchers took 80 undergraduate students who reported having chronic stress over the previous months. They heard words of affirmation before they completed 30 difficult associated problem-solving items under time pressure, which basically means they took a test. The students who were affirmed (or encouraged) demonstrated improved problem-solving performance. The control group underperformed.

Don Miguel Ruiz furthered the conversation surrounding words of affirmation in his book *The Four Agreements* by characterizing the importance of being impeccable with your words. The idea behind this agreement is that your words are powerful and can create and manifest reality, both for yourself and for others. Therefore, it's essential to use your words wisely and with integrity.

Being impeccable with your words means speaking with truth, kindness, and respect. It means avoiding gossip, rumors, and negativity and refraining from using words to harm or manipulate others. It also means being true to yourself and speaking your own truth without fear or hesitation.

When you are impeccable with your words, you create a positive energy and environment around you. Your words have the power to heal, to inspire, and to uplift others. They can also help you create the life you want by affirming your goals and intentions and by expressing gratitude for what you already have.

Overall, being impeccable with your words is a powerful practice that can bring you greater happiness, success, and fulfillment in life.

The concept surrounding the power of words of affirmation can be summarized in the Pygmalion Effect. The Pygmalion Effect, also known as the self-fulfilling prophecy, is a psychological phenomenon in which higher expectations lead to improved performance. It is named after Pygmalion, a character in Greek mythology who fell in love with a statue he had carved, and his love brought it to life.

In the context of human behavior, the Pygmalion Effect refers to the idea that when people are treated as if they can achieve great things, they are more likely to do so. This happens because people internalize the expectations that others have for them, and this internalization motivates them to work harder and perform better.

The Pygmalion Effect is often seen in educational and workplace settings. For example, if a teacher expects certain students to excel, they are more likely to provide them with extra attention, feedback, and opportunities for growth, which in turn can improve the students' performance. Similarly, if a manager expects their employees to perform well, they are more likely to provide them with the resources and support they need to do so.

On the other hand, if people are treated as if they are not capable of performing well, they are more likely to internalize those expectations and perform poorly. This is known as the Golem Effect, which is the opposite of the Pygmalion Effect.

Findings confirmed that the sympathetic nervous system responses to stressors is reduced by self-affirmation. People who are affirmed, either through self-affirmation or others affirming and instilling confidence in them, performed better and dealt with life stressors in healthier ways.

My father was a master of the Pygmalion Effect. He constantly spoke words of affirmation to my siblings and me. He gave us the confidence not only that we could succeed but that we could be great.

The power of this love language to impact the heart was demonstrated in a study in which researchers in the UK looked at psychological characteristics of over 8,000 people and found that those who scored high on optimism (similar to words of affirmation in that both focus on the positive aspects of life and encourage individuals to adopt a positive mindset) and a sense of well-being enjoyed a 30% lower risk of developing heart disease. Other studies report similar findings: In a study of over 70,000 women followed for over 10 years, those who scored highest on an optimism questionnaire had a significantly lower risk of death from heart attacks (38%) and strokes (39%).

Acts of Service and the Heart

Love is a verb in action, as emphasized in 1 Corinthians 13:4-7, a passage from one of the world's oldest texts, the Bible. Here, love is characterized as being "patient, kind, not envious, boastful, or proud. It does not dishonor others, is not self-centered, is not easily provoked, and forgives without holding grudges." In essence, love is a verb that involves actively demonstrating these qualities in our interactions with others. In a previous discussion, we also mentioned one of the Greek words for love: *agape*. *Agape* represents empathy, altruism, volunteering, and giving, regardless of an individual's relationship with another person.

Studies show that volunteering reduces stress and increases positive and relaxed feelings by releasing dopamine. Volunteers report that spending time with others in service provides them with a sense of meaning and appreciation. Both giving and receiving have a stress reducing effect.

A Carnegie Mellon study looked at those who volunteered 200 hours a year and found the higher the volunteer hours, the lower the blood pressure levels. Other studies found health benefits resulting from as little as 100 hours of volunteering per year, or just under two hours a week.

Another study published in *The Journal of Happiness* examined over 70,000 individuals in the United Kingdom. Participants were questioned about their volunteering habits and mental health, distress, and functioning in everyday life. Participants were surveyed every two years from 1996 until 2014. Findings revealed that people who volunteered within the prior year were more satisfied with their lives and benefited from better overall health than non-volunteers. Researchers also found that the more the person volunteered, the greater the benefits. It's common sense; the more one puts into something, the more they get out of it.

A study conducted in 2020 with middle-aged people found the association between daily stressors and negative effects were weaker on the days the participants volunteered. This is a powerful statistic because this is during a person's most productive years. This is when people raise children and help their parents. One would think that giving more time would stress busy people out, but instead, giving actually relieved their stress. The researchers concluded that volunteering created a stress-buffering effect that contributed to improved emotional well-being for individuals who volunteered on a regular basis. It's simple: The more you give, the more you receive.

Physical Touch

Michelangelo said, "To touch is to give life." Those words spoken some five hundred years ago still hold true today. The COVID-19 pandemic took away physical touch and life. Many people had to forgo physical touch with friends and loved ones, which has been challenging and difficult for many. This has been especially hard for people who rely on physical touch as a primary way of expressing and receiving love and affection. The lack of physical touch and social isolation during the pandemic has also led to increased feelings of loneliness, anxiety, and depression for many people. This highlights the importance of physical touch in promoting emotional well-being and social connection.

Studies have found that various forms of physical touch can increase oxytocin levels in the brain, including hugs, handholding, massage, and even petting an animal. It's been suggested that oxytocin can even be released when exposed to certain types of sound and light. This indicates that there is a positive interaction between touch and psychological support and that touch is health promoting. In other studies, hugs have been shown to decrease the release of cortisol, the stress hormone, and to lower blood pressure and heart rate during stressful situations.

Do you ever instinctively reach out to hug someone that is emotionally distraught? Human connectedness is powerful. I recall the many moments of disappointment in life when a hug from my parents, my siblings, my kids, and my wife made me feel better. I wasn't aware of how it made me feel better, I only knew it did. Physical touch is so powerful that research has even shown that hugs can strengthen the immune system.

Let's look at a study that examined individuals' susceptibility to infectious disease. In this study, researchers looked at how stress from relationships, the support people receive, and hugs could affect the likelihood of getting sick when exposed to viruses. They found that stress and lack of support were linked to a higher chance of getting infected after being exposed to a virus. However, people who felt supported and received hugs more frequently were less likely to get sick. Hugs seemed to help both by reducing the chances of getting infected and by making illness symptoms less severe. This shows that physical touch, like hugging, could play a role in protecting against getting sick.

Other research has suggested that oxytocin may play a role in the beneficial effects of physical touch on health and well-being, even pain.

A 2020 study from Germany's Brewer University Ruhr put couples between the ages of 19 and 32 through a stress-inducing experiment. Scientists hypothesized that hugging would decrease the production of cortisol in the body's stress response. Half of the group hugged their partners for 20 seconds before placing their hands in ice water, while the other couples did not hug before putting their hands in the ice water. Participants held their hands in the water for three minutes. Researchers surveyed participants' mood and measured blood pressure and cortisol levels before and 25 minutes after the test. The results? Women who hugged their partners before the experiment were able to tolerate pain better and had lower levels of cortisol afterward compared to the control group. Just think, receiving a hug before a stressful event or during one can give you superpowers to resist pain and mitigate the stress hormone cascade that leads to Broken Heart Syndrome and other diseases.

Why the Five Love Languages Matter

Understanding the five love languages brings it home to us that love is more than a feeling. Long before I heard of Gary Chapman's book, *The Five Love Languages,* I *lived* the five love languages. I tell people I was a pleasant surprise. I was an unexpected gift rather than a planned event. As a result, my five siblings' ages range from 16 years older to 3 years older than me. Six in the house made for an interesting childhood. My loving parents raised us, but my eldest siblings almost took over a parental role when I was young. As a result, I had more parents than most. Each brought with them their special gifts and perspectives. As I reminisce, I recall my father's unflinching belief in me. He fed my soul with words of affirmation. My dad wasn't a prophet, but he prophesied my success. Much to my chagrin, I would overhear my dad saying, "My son is going to be a doctor." At the time I was embarrassed, but now I realize what he was doing. Though some might call that boasting or bragging, my dad was planting the seeds of success—the seeds of love—in me and all his kids. He was being intentional or *impeccable with his words* like Don Luis Miguel wrote about in *The Four Agreements*. He sang our praises. "My children are brilliant. They're the smartest kids in the world. They're going to accomplish big things in life." Dad liberally sowed these seeds throughout my childhood, teen, and early adult years. His words of affirmation played a role in building my foundation, and with that solid foundation, I have been blessed to achieve my goals. It was like my father willed me into who I am today, and it was good-will.

My mother embodied the spirit of philanthropy, albeit in unconventional ways. Instead of traditional monetary contributions, she enriched the souls of our family and community with her boundless love and selfless service. Hosting cooking classes and eagerly volunteering her time were just a glimpse of her compassionate nature. Amid her myriad responsibilities, Mom never overlooked her children's needs, ensuring we were well fed and clothed. She extended her kindness to the lonely and those in need, often sacrificing her own desires for our well-being. While our family wasn't affluent, we always had enough, and my parents even managed to send us to private school. Her life serves as a living testament to love, and though our family was its primary beneficiary, she had abundant love to share with the community through bible studies, culinary expertise, and a comforting shoulder for anyone in need. Even at the age of 88 (apologies, Mom, for revealing your age), she continues to volunteer while making sure I lack nothing, ensuring that my favorite dishes are on the table and, of course, showering me with boundless love and unwavering support.

One of the greatest acts of love my parents demonstrated was when they adopted a teenager from our church when they were in their 50s. The young teen was a family friend and was in a situation where she would have to be moved to a group home. Their generosity allowed her to live in a loving home. They saved her from bad influences. It was pure altruism. They weren't looking for recognition. They never planned on having another child, but they felt compelled to open their home and share whatever resources they had to support and cherish another soul. That's love in action. That's *agape*.

Why is it important that love is an action word? Because it has the power to change lives. When Gary Chapman summarized my life's lessons and modernized the Greek perspective on love in his *Five Languages of Love*, he spoke about the words of affirmation I received from my father. Chapman spoke about the quality time I received from my siblings. He spoke about the giving and receiving of gifts that my father so eloquently demonstrated. He spoke about the acts of service that my mother performed. He spoke about the physical touch that my family demonstrated. He spoke about the bonding power of these acts. When Chapman talked about the Greek term *philia*, which is brotherly love, *storge,* or familial love, and *agape* love, which is altruistic love, he brought to us an understanding that these were the foundations that sustained love in relationships throughout our lives.

I believe that my parents' love, which they liberally offered through their forgiveness and encouragement, gave me the confidence and resiliency I needed to become an interventional cardiologist. Their unconditional love and support lives within me and guides the way I parent my children. I know from the depths of my heart that without their legacy of love, I would not have the courage to place wires and balloons down the arteries of thousands of hearts. My parents' investment of time and love, given to me during my formative years, reaped astounding dividends in my life and my career.

The Love Hormone and Stress

My life and perspective on life changed dramatically after my kids were born. I remember those early years learning how to parent and watching how my wife was so patient and caring when the kids were sick or irritable. I remember how she would cuddle them close to her in her bosom and rock them to sleep (although sometimes she fell asleep first). The peace that transcended over her face and theirs was angelic. Scientists have uncovered that the calming effect I witnessed in my wife and kids during those moments was triggered by a hormone called oxytocin.

Oxytocin is a powerful hormone or, as I like to say, a body messenger. It is often described as the love hormone and the anti-stress hormone. Oxytocin counteracts the effects of stress by reducing blood pressure and cortisol levels. It increases pain thresholds and exerts an anxiety-killing effect. Oxytocin is secreted during bonding. Examples include my experience watching my wife with my kids or hand holding during date night. It is often referred to as the bonding hormone as well as the cuddling hormone. Oxytocin causes people to seek relationships, meaningful discussions, and social interactions with one another. Oxytocin is the antithesis of stress.

Stress makes the heart work harder, but oxytocin neutralizes the harmful effects of stress. I mentioned before how stress can cause your vessels to constrict. Studies show that higher plasma oxytocin levels are associated with greater dilation of the vessels and decreased heart rate. This improves heart functionality by decreasing the force that the heart muscle needs to contract. Oxytocin also reduces the effects of stress on the gastrointestinal system by increasing muscle contractions, which allows acid to leave the stomach.

Forgiveness and the Heart

Anyone who has loved or cared for someone in their life knows that love takes effort. My parents were masters of forgiveness, at least when it came to my siblings and myself. I remember about six months after I got my driver's license, I got into not one but two fender benders that were my fault for not paying attention. The crazy part was that I wasn't grounded. My parents didn't take my keys. There were no harsh words or reprimands. I only remember my dad handing me the keys and telling me he forgave me when I said I was sorry and admitted I wasn't paying attention. Their primary concern was for my safety.

Forgiveness is love in action. Forgiveness isn't just for the person who has wronged you, it is for you. Forgiveness is closely related to stress. When we hold on to anger, resentment, or other negative emotions toward someone who has wronged us, it can create a lot of stress and tension in our lives. This can lead to chronic stress, which can have negative impacts on our physical and mental health over time.

Forgiveness is a superpower because it is a stress buster, which makes it one of the key components in health and well-being. To prove this theory, researchers have conducted many studies to validate the power of forgiveness in our lives. An April 2016 study, published in *The Annals of Behavioral Medicine*, included 300 individuals who ranged from teenagers to age 79. Results were the same in all age groups. People who forgave experienced a decrease in their perception of their stress.

A study published in the *Journal of Behavioral Medicine* examined forgiveness as a predictor of mortality (death). This study revealed a significant relationship between forgiving and decreased risk of overall all causes of death.

This next study looked at the power of forgiveness to heal a broken heart. Researchers performed a myocardial perfusion scan (an imaging study that looks at the amount of blood flow to various regions of the heart) on 17 patients who had documented lack of blood flow to portions of the heart with anger recall. The 17 individuals were divided into two groups. One group received an intervention of 10 weeks of interpersonal forgiveness sessions, and the other group, the control group, saw a psychologist. After the ten-week period, retesting showed that the forgiveness group had fewer anger recalled perfusion defects. Simply put, they showed more blood flow to their heart muscle. They also made significant gains in their ability to forgive. The researchers concluded that forgiveness intervention is an effective means of reducing anger-induced blood flow defects to the heart muscles in coronary artery disease patients.

Forgiveness allows us to let go of self-defeating anger. It is not about letting others off the hook; it is about divesting ourselves from the hurt and pain of holding on to anger or fear. Forgiving does not mean that someone who harms us will not go to jail, it means that we let go of ideas of revenge and anger in order to free ourselves. We don't need to go to prison with the person who harmed us. When we hold grudges or even justifiable upsets, we imprison our hearts. At some point, for our own well-being, we must let it go. It is said that forgiveness is the best gift that you can give to yourself.

Gratitude and Health

Throughout my life, it was apparent how my father influenced a room by his presence, his smile, and his energy. But his greatest power was his expression of gratitude. He could make even the smallest gift seem as if it were a winning lottery ticket. He had the knack of making you feel as if you were the greatest gift giver in the entire world. He had an extraordinary gift, the gift of gratitude. Even toward the end of his life, when he had every right to be depressed and sad, or cantankerous, he continued to give his greatest gift—gratitude. He could hardly see, he couldn't walk, and he had a diabetic foot ulcer, but he was still grateful for the small things. When I stopped by to feed him or talk with him, he would smile brightly and talk about how blessed he was. He talked about how the sun shone brightly and how much he loved his family. He would joke about how he was trying to be just like me, and when I left, he always hugged me. I remember his touch.

Gratitude is another superpower. Gratitude is love in action. The higher our stress, the poorer our health. Gratitude has the ability to neutralize stress. Gratitude impacts the resiliency that bolsters health. Let's look at gratitude's overall impact. Studies show that gratitude is associated with higher levels of our good cholesterol. The bloodstream hosts good and bad cholesterol. I describe bad cholesterol like a criminal lurking in neighborhoods looking for opportunities to vandalize. Think of your good cholesterol as police officers patrolling and trying to lock up the bad cholesterol criminals. The more police officers you have, the healthier the community. The community is the vascular system. Studies show that gratitude is associated with higher levels of good cholesterol and lower levels of bad cholesterol.

And if that's not enough to make you stop and think or at least stop and be grateful, there's more. Gratitude is associated with lowered blood pressure in the face of stress.

Researchers have correlated gratitude with other markers of heart health. One such marker is heart rate variability (HRV). HRV is the variation in the time between each beat of the heart. HRV is closely related to stress. When a person experiences stress, their body's natural fight or flight response is activated, which causes an increase in heart rate and a decrease in HRV. This is because stress activates the sympathetic nervous system (SNS), which is responsible for preparing the body for action in response to stressors. A normal HRV is a marker of being calm and a state of harmony in the nervous system. HRV is associated with stress and mental clarity.

The research on the effects of gratitude on human health has demonstrated beneficial effects on mental health, kidney function, inflammation, diabetes mellitus, sleep quality, and the relaxing of the lining of vessels called the endothelium.

A 2015 study published in the *Journal of Happiness Studies* discovered that elderly participants who undertook a two-week gratitude intervention experienced an increase in well-being, leading to improved social functioning and decreased perceived stress. Similarly, a 2004 study conducted by McCraty found that participants who practiced gratitude exhibited reduced levels of the stress hormone cortisol, resulting in improved cardiac functioning and resilience from negative experiences. Numerous studies have demonstrated that practicing gratitude can help individuals better manage stress compared to those who do not engage in gratitude practices. By appreciating and acknowledging the small things in life, individuals can retrain their brains to approach their present circumstances with a broader perspective and heightened awareness. Practicing gratitude can also benefit healthcare practitioners who are experiencing burnout, with one study finding that keeping a gratitude journal for two weeks led to a 28% reduction in perceived stress and a 16% reduction in depression. During the pandemic, when empathy and compassion fatigue had been particularly high, studies suggested gratitude helped offset stress by reducing stress hormone levels by as much as 23%.

Healthy Heart Doc Tips on How to Love

When Angie said love doesn't exist, it struck a chord. Even though she understood the concept that love is a verb, it didn't remove the pain that she experienced, the hurt, or the loneliness, but it did provide a new perspective. Angie needed more than what intellect could offer. She needed easy-to-follow instructions on how to make love come alive in her life. "Angie, I know your hurt is real, but in order to move past the pain, you must heal. You must love again."

At this point, Angie was on board. She recognized the truth—her life and health depended on making life-altering changes. She had to move past her pain and into her love. Angie committed to a six-week building love challenge. I felt relieved when she saw the light and was warmed to see love taking action in her life. Angie completed the six-week challenge and as a result of her actions, she built that invaluable resiliency needed to combat stress. Love in action was her mighty companion. Her health improved. Magic? No, but the results of taking daily actions are magical. That's why I want to share ideas that can improve your life, your health, and your relationships.

We start with SMART goals. A SMART goal is specific. It can be accomplished within a certain time frame, and it is measurable. If you want to spark the magic in your life and change your world, here's a road map.

Take the Gratitude Challenge

1. Get a gratitude journal and keep it handy.

One hour before bedtime, write down one thing you're grateful for. Simple, easy, measurable, and achievable. The power of gratitude is a manifestation of love. We meet the goal of being time-based by doing this for one hour before bedtime for six weeks. The second week, write two things you are grateful for. The third week, write down three things you are thankful for and for the remaining weeks, write down four things you are grateful for.

2. Say, "Thank You"

- Develop a habit of saying thank you for expected service, such as to your food server or the one who brings you coffee.

- Be sure to say thank you for unexpected service, such as someone holding the door for you.

- Say thank you when someone lets you in a line. This should be a slam dunk for most people, but if you are not offering gratitude for these little things, your thank you muscle is too weak.

- Put down that cell phone and say thank you to the checkout clerk

- Say thank you to your spouse for cooking, cleaning, bill paying, earning money so you can go to school, or for whatever service they provide. Say thank you to those closest to you, and say it often.

- Write personal thank you notes to people. This is especially effective at work. People work harder for *praises* than raises. Though we don't offer gratitude in order to be repaid, this idea, that people value appreciation more than money, reminds us of the power of gratitude.

3. Perform Random Acts of Kindness

The world is built on kindness. When Oprah Winfrey started her random acts of kindness program in 2015, she opened the hearts of millions and made the world a better place. Being kind to people is the gift that gives twice because when we give to others, we give to ourselves. Remember how good it feels to give. Be intentional about your random acts of kindness. Here are some suggestions of random, unsolicited acts of kindness:

- Open the door for someone.

- Pick up trash as you walk.

- Put a coin in an expired parking meter.

- Send flowers to a friend for no reason at all.

- Get in touch with somebody that had an impact on your life and tell them how much their guidance or attention meant to you.

- Offer someone 100% of your attention when they are speaking to you.

4. Affirm Others

Practice saying something positive to everyone you encounter. Be sensitive with this one. If someone is grieving, the best thing we can say to them is, "I'm here. I am so sorry you are going through this." We dont want to spout platitudes about how God doesn't give you more than you can handle. Again, something such as, "It's going to take time, and I am here to listen", is a positive in this situation. If someone looks haggard, look for the thing about them that looks good, or point out a quality you admire. "I've always admired your tenacity." Or "Your light seems to shine even on the darkest of days." Be sure to include yourself when handing out compliments or life-affirming words. The most affirming words we can say to anyone is, "I love you." How about a shout-out when you look in the mirror each morning: "I love you."

5. Forgive:

Start with yourself. Write down everything you think you have done to harm yourself or others. Make amends with those you can by offering an apology or making retribution when appropriate. Offer apologies to yourself for the times you have not taken care of yourself. Journal about the events or experiences that bind you to the past. Writing it out is like having a personal therapist. Start writing about the event or situation and how upset you are. Hold nothing back. Keep writing until you are not so triggered by the event or situation. No hurry. You might write a daily page for a month before you feel like you can let go. Write down all the reasons you can't forgive yourself and offer these reasons up to God or to a Higher Power. Ask God or your higher power to help you forgive. Your prayer might be something like, "Even though I do not know if I can forgive, I am willing to forgive. Help me." When you feel complete in the process, write across each page, "Paid in full. I forgive myself."

Next, work with every event, situation, or person that you need to forgive. Tailor the process above to fit your needs.

Hopefully I've convinced you of the power of love and its impact on your health and well-being. Using the ideas and taking the challenges I've offered in this chapter will change your life. Now is the time for you to take action. It's up to you. For additional tips on integrating love into your life to alleviate stress and foster emotional healing, connect with our community at www.DrBatiste.com.

CHAPTER 5

Food

Angie was experiencing multiple challenges that were taking a toll on her well-being. The pandemic of 2020-2022, the loss of her mother, her broken relationship, and the empty nest syndrome were all contributing factors that led to her diagnosis of Broken Heart Syndrome. This was the tipping point for Angie, as the cumulative effect of these stressors became too much for her to bear. She realized that the demands in her life were exceeding her available resources.

To cope with the overwhelming stress, Angie turned to what can be described as "fake resources." These are temporary solutions that people often turn to in the hopes of alleviating their mental anguish, but they ultimately leave them feeling even emptier. While some may turn to cigars, cigarettes, alcohol, or drugs as fake resources, Angie found comfort in an old friend from her childhood— food.

It's worth noting that there is a stigma attached to some fake resources, which may have deterred Angie from indulging in them. However, comfort food was a familiar and accessible option that she could turn to.

Angie's relationship with food was complex, much like it is for many of us. The question of whether nature (genetics) or nurture (environment) shapes the way we respond to life's stressors is a source of curiosity for many. Researchers have discovered that genetics can play a role in stress-coping behaviors. Some people may be genetically predisposed to handle stress better than others due to their genetic makeup.

For instance, specific genes may influence how the brain processes stress, including the regulation of stress hormones such as cortisol. In addition, genetic variations may impact the expression of genes involved in stress responses, leading to differences in how individuals respond to stress. However, it's important to note that genetics is just one aspect of stress-coping behaviors.

The environment also plays a crucial role in stress-coping behaviors. Studies have shown that early life experiences, such as childhood trauma or adverse events, can have long-term effects on an individual's stress response system. These effects include changes in stress hormone levels, brain function, and an individual's behavior.

Looking back on her life, Angie realized that her stress-response relationship with food was mostly influenced by her upbringing. During her childhood, she learned by example to associate refined foods that were high in salt, sugar, and fat with happy occasions like birthdays and holidays. Angie recalled when she was sad growing up how her mom would make her favorite treats or take her on special outings, treating her to donuts, ice cream, or pizza to make her feel better. These lessons from her childhood became a strong foundation for her, providing her with a "resource" that she could rely on during times of stress in her adult life.

As she grew older, Angie found herself relying on this resource more and more. Given her mindset, which is shared by many, it was predictable that when she faced the challenges of COVID, along with the loss of loved ones and relationships, she turned once again to her old companion and false resource: comfort food. This situation is reminiscent of the movie *Castaway* with Tom Hanks, where he was stranded on a deserted island and personified a volleyball named Wilson as his sole companion and friend, providing him with a sense of support—a sort of fake resource—to help him cope with stressful moments.

It was Ann Wigmore who once said, "Food can either be the most powerful form of medicine or the slowest form of poison." This means that food can either be a real resource or a fake one. Through my experiences as a physician and my research on the effects of nutrition, I have come to believe that food plays a crucial role in our overall health, and this can be summarized by the health equation: Health = Resiliency/Stress. The right nutrition can increase our resiliency, while the wrong nutrition can add to our stress levels.

While I am now a passionate advocate for plant-based nutrition and lifestyle practices, this hasn't always been the case. At first, I was hesitant to share the power of nutrition with my patients, fearing that I would be seen as different and possibly ostracized. Additionally, I wondered if the nutrition research was too good to be true.

I soon realized that the lack of emphasis on nutrition and lifestyle practices in medical education and board certification exams was the root of the problem. I came to understand that resources go where value is placed, and unfortunately, in the medical field, value is placed on passing exams that focus on pharmaceuticals, procedures, and predetermined quality metrics that do not include nutrition and lifestyle. This means that nutrition and lifestyle practices are often not prioritized.

Despite my initial apprehension, life events pushed me to share the power of nutrition with my patients. After seeing dramatic improvements in the health of the first three patients that I shared this information with, I was fully committed to incorporating nutrition and lifestyle practices into my medical practice. Looking back, I recall reading the wise words of Dr. David Sackett, who said that half of what you learn in medical school will eventually be shown to be either dead wrong or out of date. This is why it's so important to know how to learn and critically appraise the literature.

Thanks to my medical education, residency, and fellowship training, I've developed the tools I need to learn and stay up-to-date on the latest research. I'm excited to share this knowledge with you and empower you to take control of your health through nutrition and lifestyle practices. In this chapter, we'll explore not only how stress affects our diet but also how our diets impact our perception of stress and overall health. My hope is that this information will inspire and empower you on your journey toward better health.

Comfort Foods and a Broken Heart

As night fell, Angie's emotional walls crumbled and tears streamed down her face. She had hit rock bottom, and only memories of the comfort foods she had shared with her mother and husband brought her solace. It's no surprise that scientists have found that our food preferences change after a breakup or loss of a loved one due to the stress hormone cortisol. Emotional stress can be overwhelming, activating the amygdala, which plays a crucial role in processing emotions and generating responses to perceived threats. This cascade of events triggers our bodies to release cortisol and prepares us for action, but when we don't need to run or fight, we are left with a flood of hormones that can impact our food choices.

Comfort food can have the temporary effect of decreasing stress and anxiety due to the emotional connection and psychological association we have with certain foods. Comfort food is often associated with positive memories and emotions, and eating these foods can trigger feelings of nostalgia, happiness, and comfort. These feelings can provide a brief distraction from stress and anxiety and may help improve our mood in the short term.

Cortisol increases blood glucose levels, which can cause cravings for sugary or high-carbohydrate foods, leading to a cycle of fluctuating blood glucose levels and hunger. Stress can also lead to an increased consumption of high fat, high sugar foods, which can activate brain pathways similar to drugs and affect our preferences and cravings for them. Comfort foods can increase the brain chemical serotonin. Serotonin is known to regulate mood and promote feelings of calmness and well-being, which may help alleviate stress and anxiety. While these foods may initially provide temporary relief, the benefits are short-lived and can lead to repetitive consumption.

Researchers have found that a diet rich in carbohydrates promotes an increase in insulin production, which decreases competing amino acids. This makes it easier for tryptophan to cross the blood-brain barrier, increasing serotonin levels in the brain and decreasing feelings of helplessness, depression, loss of control, and distress. Similarly, Dallman's study suggests that people eat comfort food to reduce anxiety, but this type of symptom relief can be problematic in the long run.

Why Can't I Stop Eating Certain Foods?

Angie's weight gain didn't happen overnight, just like her reliance on food for comfort did not happen overnight. Her use of food as a coping mechanism had progressed from occasional to frequent and from frequent to daily. Angie admitted that when she tried to stop eating the food that comforted her, her mood would spiral and she would become irritable. It is said that art imitates life, and in 2010, Mars Wrigley Confectionery launched an artistic ad campaign: "You're not you when you're hungry." The ad depicted mood changes being alleviated only by taking a bite of a Snickers candy bar. This commercial was an example of effective advertising, as it portrayed the idea that food can change one's mood. Whether it was art imitating Angie's life or Angie's life imitating art, Angie's cravings for comfort food started to consume her. The cravings would often arise at any time, from work hours to midnight trips to a 24-hour gas station. Although Angie did not frequently weigh herself, her weight gain became noticeable through her clothing, and her ability to perform basic activities during daily living was impacted.

Angie came to my office feeling hopeless about her inability to stop consuming comfort foods. As I listened to her, my mind recalled my past thoughts of arrogance when I had heard someone say they were addicted to chocolate. I had believed that it was simply a matter of making better choices and had dismissed the idea of food addiction. However, addiction is defined as a lack of control over usage, social impairment, and craving and can cause harm to relationships and interfere with work or school obligations. People with addiction may continue the behavior despite harm and may develop a tolerance over time. Angie's relationship with food had entered the realm of addiction, characterized by her lack of control, intense cravings, hidden consumption, and prioritization of fulfilling the craving despite other obligations.

Research has shown that food cravings involve the same areas of the brain as drug addiction, with similar neurotransmitters involved and many identical symptoms. Certain foods, particularly junk foods like candy, sugary sodas, and fried foods, can have a powerful effect on the performance centers of the brain. These effects are caused by neurotransmitters like dopamine.

During our session, Angie expressed frustration at her perceived lack of willpower. I explained to her that whether we called it "willpower," "cravings," or "addiction," her relationship with food had become unhealthy. I reassured her that her struggle with food was not a matter of willpower but rather a complex issue triggered by dopamine signals that created a physical and chemical transformation in her body.

The concept of food cravings/addiction is described as the dietary pleasure trap in *The Pleasure Trap*, a book by Douglas J. Lisle and Alan Goldhamer. In this book, Drs. Lisle and Goldhamer explain that the main driver of human behavior is the motivation to conserve energy, seek pleasure, and avoid pain. The dietary pleasure trap arises from a mismatch between our natural psychology and the modern food environment, making us vulnerable to excessive dietary and lifestyle choices. This system of forces, due to the motivational triad (conserve energy, seek pleasure, and avoid pain), can be challenging to escape from.

Our activities as humans are pursued through the lens of the motivational triad. We often gravitate toward the path of least resistance, which can involve consuming "convenience" foods that require minimal thought, expense, or effort. While this preference aligns with our energy conservation programming, our pursuit of pleasure, and our avoidance of pain, it can lead to obesity, exhaustion, and addiction (the pleasure trap).

The dietary pleasure trap is composed of five phases. The first phase pertains to the brain's reaction when we consume everyday healthy foods such as fruits and vegetables. These are the foods that our bodies are designed to eat, and we experience mild elevation of dopamine upon consuming them. We derive enjoyment from these foods, but they do not induce lethargy or intense cravings.

The second phase occurs when we eat processed foods, which are devoid of fiber, minerals, and vitamins but are rich in salt, sugar, and fat. I always describe the food as "It melts in your mouth, not in your hand." It's like pre-chewed food. These foods are easy to digest and provide a higher assimilable calorie intake per bite, leading to the brain releasing higher doses of dopamine. This creates a "drug-like" effect, causing us to crave and consume more of these foods. After consuming large amounts of these comfort foods, our energy levels drop, and we feel lethargic and relaxed. Ultra-processed or refined foods can even decrease pain, which is why doctors give infants sugar water before circumcision.

In the third phase of the pleasure trap, the brain tries to defend itself against this high stimulus of dopamine by dulling the sensation. We experience this when the first bite of cake tastes amazing but subsequent bites become less phenomenal. We enter a search and explore phase looking for that "first love." To achieve the same satisfaction, we must consume richer and richer foods, which can lead to more medical problems.

Am I the Only One Who Has This Problem With Food?

Absolutely not! The pandemic of 2020 really exposed America's susceptibility to stress and its use of food for comfort. A study published in 2022 Nutrients Journal surveyed over 3,900 adults and found increases in the consumption of junk food with over 59% of adults consuming unhealthy snacks/desserts and over a third consuming sugar sweetened beverages during the stress-filled pandemic of 2020. The Stress in America organization conducts a yearly survey focusing on a different subject as it relates to stress. In 2022, the focus was on the influences of stress on our eating patterns. The survey found that 38% of adults surveyed said they'd overeaten or eaten unhealthy foods in the past month because of stress. Half of the adults reported engaging in these behaviors weekly or more often; 33% said they overate or ate poorly because it helped distract them from their stress; 27% of the last group surveyed said they ate to manage stress; and 34% said this behavior was a habit.

There is a common assumption that physicians are better at coping with stress than the general population because of their medical training and experience. While it is true that physicians receive training on how to manage stress and maintain their well-being, this does not mean that they are immune to the negative effects of stress.

In fact, the medical profession is known to be highly stressful, and physicians are at risk of experiencing burnout, depression, anxiety, and other mental health issues as a result. The demands of the job, such as long work hours, high pressure, and exposure to traumatic events, can take a toll on a physician's mental and emotional health.

Medscape surveyed physicians experiencing burnout (a form of stress) and found 35% cope by eating junk food.

The prevalence of overeating and consuming unhealthy foods is widespread, with many of us starting these poor eating habits during early childhood and continuing them into adulthood. Unfortunately, our habits are often reinforced by the pervasive images we see in the media, including on television.

In fact, a recent study published in the *International Journal of Disease Reversal and Prevention* (2021) found that a staggering 58% of commercials advertised fast food chains, with an average of 3.1 more unhealthy items promoted than healthy ones. Furthermore, during the pandemic, Penn State researchers discovered that live-streaming ads targeting online gamers for alcohol and junk food had increased.

According to the Rudd Center for Food Policy and Health at the University of Connecticut, their research indicates that candy, sugary drinks, snacks, and cereals represented a significant majority (three-quarters) of Spanish-language and Black-targeted TV ad spending in 2021, an increase from 2017. These junk food and marketing industries continue to thrive, while our health suffers as a result.

Eating Trends in the United States

The United States is the bearer of the standard American diet. More than 70% of packaged foods in the United States are classified as ultra-processed food and represent approximately

60% of all calories consumed by Americans. The Center for Disease Control discovered that more than 1/3 of American adults eat drive-thru food on a daily basis. Amongst those who eat ultra-processed foods, studies estimate the percentage of food eaten from ready-to-eat and mixed dishes increased from 2.2% to 11.2%. The consumption of sweets had increased from 10.7% to 12.9%.

One of my most vivid memories of my dad was his love for fast food, whether it was from the rapidly expanding fast food restaurants that dotted our neighborhoods or the ready-to-eat meals and snacks sold in convenience stores, such as TV dinners, ice cream, candy, and chips. Going grocery shopping with my dad was always a treat because my siblings and I knew we would get the goodies we wanted. I remember how we would excitedly display our purchases on the dining room table, only to have my mom shake her head in disapproval as she peeked under the pile of treats to ensure that we had also bought the "ingredients" for two weeks of healthy meals. I encountered duality in my food experience, as my dad was also particular about the quality of fruits and vegetables he bought. Despite purchasing processed foods locally in our Compton neighborhood, my dad would intentionally drive 10-15 miles to a grocery store in a different city where the produce was of a magical quality, as if they had been picked directly from the Garden of Eden. Looking back now, I realize that I lived in a food swamp and a food desert (some call this an apartheid state to infer an intentional process as opposed to a natural phenomenon). The local grocer sold poor-quality fruits and vegetables alongside ultra-processed foods. For those lacking access to transportation, they had to rely on liquor or convenience stores, with the ice cream truck serving as an early version of Grubhub or Postmates, delivering these tempting treats directly to our doorstep. To this day, I can vividly recall the melodies emanating from those ice cream trucks, as if the tunes were playing just yesterday.

Food deserts refer to geographic areas that lack access to

health-promoting foods, while food swamps are areas with an overabundance of fast food restaurants and junk food. Together, these conditions contribute to an environment of nutritional stress and food insecurity, meaning that people in these communities lack access to nutritious foods. Studies have shown that high levels of food insecurity are associated with increased consumption of ultra-processed foods, and that adults who are food-insecure or who receive Supplemental Nutrition Assistance Program (SNAP) benefits have a higher consumption of ultra-processed foods. This may help explain the diet-related health disparities observed in these populations.

A 2022 study reported a significant increase in calorie intake from ultra-processed foods, particularly among the non-Hispanic Black community, where consumption increased from 62% to 72.5%. Mexican American youths' consumption of processed foods also increased from 55.8% to 63.5% compared to non-Hispanic whites. The burden of consumption of ultra-processed foods falls disproportionately on communities of color, which tend to have food deserts and swamps. A 2016 survey by McKinsey & Company found that one out of every five African American households was situated in a food desert with limited access to grocery stores, restaurants, or farmers markets.

Research suggests that the foods sold in convenience stores and fast food establishments are linked to chronic disease and may contribute to the disparities in health outcomes.

The Role of the Environment in Certain Food Cravings

Our surroundings exert a significant influence on our behavior. Platforms such as social media, television, theaters, and advertisements play a pivotal role in driving our behaviors. However, it's often the subtle details within television commercials and movies that exert the most profound impact. The sound of a soda can being opened, the rustling of a bag of chips, the satisfying crunch of a chip, or the steam rising from a fresh pizza or hamburger all seep into our minds and become ingrained in our memories. These sensory cues trigger a cascade of thoughts and cravings that can completely consume us.

It's important to recognize that these images and sounds are not randomly placed on various media platforms. Fast food advertisements strategically infiltrate our TVs, movies, streaming platforms, and social media to ignite our hunger for ultra-processed foods. Subtly, yet effectively, they plant the seeds of desire within us.

After being exposed to these subtle cues, you might find yourself rummaging through the kitchen for something to eat, all the while unaware of the connection between your cravings and what you've just witnessed on television.

Disturbingly, a study conducted in the UK, which encompassed over 3,300 adolescents aged 11 to 19, underscored the consequences of such marketing strategies. Young individuals exposed to just one additional junk food advertisement per week, over the already high average of six, were found to consume an extra 350 calories' worth of food laden with salt, sugar, and fat every week. This translates to a staggering 18,000 additional calories per year.

Despite the detrimental effects on public health, the junk food and marketing industries continue to prosper unabated.

A study published in *The Archives of Internal Medicine* in 2011 underscored a clear correlation between how close one lives to fast food restaurants and the consumption of these foods. The allure of these foods, often laden with excessive salt, sugar, and fat, is undeniable. Research has also established a concerning link between living near fast food establishments and an increased risk of heart attacks. However, it's crucial to recognize that it's not mere proximity that elevates this risk; instead, it's the actual consumption of these foods that poses the danger.

In a separate investigation conducted by the University of

Minnesota, the consequences of fast-food consumption on heart health were quantified. The study revealed that indulging in fast food once a week amplified the risk of a heart attack by 20%. Escalating that frequency to 2 or 3 times a week correlated with a staggering 50% increase in risk, while a habit of consuming fast food four or more times weekly elevated the risk by a substantial 80%. Fast food consumption can break our hearts.

A study titled "Neighborhood Affects the Healthiness of Dietary Choices," conducted in Finland, delved into the influence of one's residential area on their dietary habits. Over a six-year period, more than 16,000 adults were scrutinized. Participants reported their eating patterns through surveys, which were then juxtaposed with national dietary recommendations. Researchers also assessed neighborhood socioeconomic status based on financial stability, educational attainment, and unemployment rates. The study illuminated a stark disparity, revealing that individuals residing in economically disadvantaged areas tended to have less healthful diets compared to their counterparts in more affluent neighborhoods.

Both health-promoting advertisements and neighborhood environments wield substantial influence over individuals' health choices. For instance, the "Miracle Food" campaign, orchestrated by the Television Bureau of Canada to prove that advertisers could sell anything, succeeded in boosting broccoli sales by a notable 8%. This achievement was attributed to the campaign's emphasis on the benefits of consuming the vegetable and its comparison to other life-changing events, such as surviving an airplane fall.

Furthermore, a 2015 study, published in BMC Public Health, brought to light the connection between neighborhoods featuring a higher concentration of healthful food outlets and elevated income levels and increased fruit and vegetable consumption.

In sum, our zip code has emerged as a significant predictor of our dietary quality, demonstrating the profound impact of both our surroundings and persuasive marketing on our food choices and, consequently, our health.

Comfort Food and Mental Health

Fast food is filled with unhealthy ingredients like excessive salt, sugar, saturated fats, trans fats, and omega-6 fatty acids, which can lead to inflammation in our bodies. Research consistently shows a link between inflammation and mental health problems such as anxiety and depression. When we choose fresh, unprocessed, and plant-based foods, our mood can become more resilient. These natural foods help our bodies absorb essential nutrients like antioxidants, omega-3 fatty acids, and fiber. Also, avoiding foods that activate the "fight or flight" stress response, such as coffee and high sugar foods can improve nutrient absorption. Research indicates that women may experience more negative emotions when consuming fast food, suggesting that it can have a stronger impact on their moods.

In a study published in *Public Health Nutrition*, individuals who frequently consumed ultra-processed foods were found to have a higher likelihood of reporting symptoms related to mental health issues. The research also unveiled some striking statistics: Those with the highest levels of ultra-processed food intake faced an 81% increased risk of reporting depression, experienced 22% more days of poor mental health per month, and encountered 19% more days of anxiety per month. Additionally, another study encompassing 8,000 adults highlighted that those men who regularly consumed approximately 16 teaspoons of sugar, equivalent to three to four regular-sized candy bars, had a 23% higher likelihood of being diagnosed with depression. Picture a different scenario where a television advertisement doesn't promote the idea that eating a candy bar can alleviate mood swings but, instead, describes how consuming such a product could potentially contribute to the onset of depression.

Excessive sugar consumption can contribute to heightened mental stress through several mechanisms. First, sugar leads to a rapid spike in blood glucose levels, providing a fleeting sensation of increased energy and alertness. However, this spike triggers the release of insulin to process the glucose, which can result in a sudden drop in blood glucose levels. This drop can cause symptoms like fatigue, irritability, and difficulty concentrating, all of which contribute to mental stress.

Secondly, excessive sugar intake has been linked to increased inflammation in the body, including in the brain. Chronic inflammation is associated with various health issues, including depression, anxiety, and cognitive decline.

In summary, excessive sugar intake can contribute to mental stress through various pathways, including blood sugar fluctuations, inflammation, addictive tendencies, and overall adverse effects on health. I can personally relate to how sugary snacks affect mood. During my childhood, my school bus dropped me off near a library where I was supposed to study. However, there was a convenience store nearby that tempted me to stray from my path and indulge in my favorite candy treats with my allowance. While the initial sugar rush provided a fleeting burst of energy, it was soon followed by a shift in my mood toward grumpiness, irritability, and inability to focus. It became clear to me, years later, that the sugar in those candies played a significant role in these mood swings. It's undeniable that the foods we consume exert a profound influence on our health, our mental well-being, and our overall perspective on life.

Nutritional Stress

The equation for health states health = resiliency/stress. Everything we do either adds to our resiliency or adds to our stress. Nutrition is no different. This led to the concept of nutritional stress. Nutritional stress is stress that's created by food's unhealthy properties. But nutritional stress is more than just eating unhealthy foods. Nutritional stress is also caused by not eating enough natural, unprocessed fiber-filled foods that are rich in vitamins, minerals, enzymes, and antioxidants. The lack of these nutrients is a major source of stress.

Types of Nutritional Stress

Food can contribute to our stress levels through various chemical processes, one of which is oxidative stress, akin to the corrosion of cars. This phenomenon also occurs within our arteries and has been linked to a range of health issues, including coronary artery disease, hypertension, diabetes, Alzheimer's Disease, and cancer.

Another form of dietary stress emerges from the consumption of foods with Advanced Glycation End Products (AGEs). AGEs result from chemical bonding between proteins and sugars or fats and sugars. To illustrate, consider the process of making a roux, a base for Cajun dishes, where flour and oil are browned together. This browning is from the Maillard reaction, which involves the bonding of fats with sugars or proteins. A similar molecular reaction occurs within our blood vessels, leading to a kind of "browning" effect. This process, in turn, contributes to vessel aging, resulting in issues like wrinkles, damage to the endothelium (the inner lining of blood vessels), diabetes, high blood pressure, and various chronic diseases.

Heterocyclic amines (HCAs) represent another source of nutritional stress. These chemicals are generated when meat, poultry, and fish are cooked at high temperatures, such as through grilling, broiling, or frying. Studies have demonstrated a connection between exposure to HCAs and an increased risk of several types of cancer, including colorectal, pancreatic, and prostate cancer. In fact, the International Agency for Research on Cancer (IARC) has classified certain HCAs as likely carcinogenic to humans.

In essence, the foods we consume can either contribute to our stress or bolster our resilience, as they engage in complex chemical reactions within our bodies, impacting our overall health and well-being.

The Role of Comfort Food in Nutritional Stress

Comfort food, fast food, and junk food contribute to oxidative stress, or what I call nutritional stress. Studies reveal that typical comfort foods create free radicals. Free radicals are unhealthy cells because they are missing something vital, an electron. Free radicals attack healthy cells, cells that are balanced and electron rich, then steal their electrons. This is similar to an unhappy child, Bobby, who may be missing his favorite lost toy dinosaur. Bobby sees Larry happily playing in the playground, and Larry has a dinosaur that looks just like the one Bobby lost. Bobby then goes after Larry and forcefully steals the dinosaur. Bobby steals his joy. Now Larry is upset and crying and unhappy. He steals a toy from Mary. Now Mary is unhappy and crying and she runs and steals a toy from Susan. The pattern continues as each unhappy child steals from another. Each child steals the others' joy. This is how free radicals act and cause cellular death.

Eating junk food, as well as exposure to various non-food toxins, triggers a series of events that result in the formation of free radicals. These free radicals initiate oxidative stress within our bodies, setting off a chain reaction of cellular damage. This oxidative stress can contribute to a range of health issues, including but not limited to cancer, high blood pressure, kidney dysfunction, vision impairment, heart disease, and numerous other illnesses.

Comfort Food and Heartbreak

Comfort food can actually harm our hearts. It's quite ironic that the very foods we turn to for comfort during tough times can lead to heart failure or a broken heart. The medical community has increasingly emphasized the crucial role of food in our overall health, especially when it comes to heart disease. In fact, a study in 2018 published in the *Journal of the American Medical Association* pointed out that nutrition was one of the top three causes of death in America, contributing to over 529,000 deaths in 2016. A staggering 84% of these deaths were linked to cardiovascular disease, with the remaining deaths attributed to cancer and diabetes. This highlights how significant our diet is in the equation of our health: Health equals our resiliency divided by our stress, and the food we eat can either add to our resiliency or contribute to our stress.

Another study looked at a typical Southern diet, which includes deep-fried foods and sugary drinks, resembling the Standard American Diet in many ways. The researchers found that following this Southern diet was associated with a higher risk of coronary heart disease. When they studied both white and black adults in different parts of the United States, they discovered that those who closely followed this Southern dietary pattern had a 72% higher risk of heart failure. Remember, Takotsubo or Broken Heart Syndrome is when the heart temporarily stops contracting properly. The Southern dietary pattern significantly increased the risk of developing heart failure by 72%. In summary, people who regularly consumed a Southern-style diet had a significantly higher risk of heart failure and even sudden cardiac death compared to those who ate the least amount of such foods.

Despite the mounting research, many people wonder if having one unhealthy meal can really make a difference. The common mindset is, "Surely, one meal won't hurt me." Well, a 2022 meta-analysis of 90 smaller studies provides an answer. It found that eating a high-fat, sugary meal can lead to abnormal functioning in the inner lining of our blood vessels called the endothelium. This lining protects our blood vessels from inflammation and blockages. The research showed that after eating a high-fat meal, the endothelium doesn't work as well as it does after eating a fiber-rich low-fat meal. So, yes, one unhealthy meal can have a negative impact. However, if you give your body time to recover and consistently eat healthy foods, it can start to heal.

To add to the evidence, a study in 2010 compared three popular diets: the Atkins diet, the South Beach Diet, and the Ornish diet. The Atkins diet, known for its low carbohydrate approach, allows meats, fish, dairy, and low-carb vegetables, making it a high-protein, high-fat diet. The South Beach Diet is a modified low-carb diet emphasizing low carbs and high-quality proteins with "healthy fats." The Ornish diet goes beyond food and promotes a comprehensive lifestyle change that includes exercise, quitting smoking, stress reduction, and transitioning to a whole-food, low-fat, plant-based diet rich in fruits, vegetables, whole grains, seeds, and legumes. Researchers studied 18 subjects who followed each of these diets sequentially, with all diets providing the same number of calories. They examined markers of inflammation, stress, and endothelial function. The results showed significant reductions in "bad cholesterol" (LDL) compared to the pre-diet baseline when participants followed the South Beach and Ornish diets. Additionally, the Ornish plan, which featured the lowest saturated fat intake, improved endothelial reactivity. These findings highlight how diet choices affect our health and can impact disease markers.

Research continues to pour in, including a study involving 12,000 patients that compared those who consumed the most ultra-processed foods with those who ate the least. Those with the highest consumption had a 66% higher likelihood of having a more advanced heart age, indicating more disease than those who consumed fewer processed foods. Other studies have shown that those who ate the most ultra-processed foods had higher than normal blood pressure, increasing their health risks. Another study with over 100,000 patients demonstrated a 12% increase in cardiovascular risks for those who consumed the most ultra-processed foods. In 2021, an article in *The Journal of the American College of Cardiology* looked at more than 3,000 healthy adults without heart disease. The study found that those who frequently consumed ultra-processed foods increased their risk of various cardiovascular diseases, including coronary artery disease and cardiovascular death.

In essence, what we eat matters a great deal for our heart health, and the evidence shows that our dietary choices can either protect or harm our cardiovascular well-being.

Comfort Food Leads to Other Health Issues

Eating comfort food leads to a multitude of health problems. Higher ultra-processed food consumption leads to an increased risk of type 2 diabetes. Each 10% caloric intake increase in ultra-processed food is associated with a 15% increased risk of type 2 diabetes. Studies associate junk food consumption with a 10% increased risk of breast cancer. Recent studies show that eating ultra-processed food puts one at increased risk for colorectal cancer.

Back to The Health Equation

Health equals resiliency divided by stress; the higher an individual's stress, the poorer an individual's health. Everything that we do adds to our resiliency or adds to our stress. When we examine this concept in the context of the Self*ish* principles, we see that each component has the ability to add to our resiliency. Higher resiliency bolsters our health. Resiliency is the process of adapting well in the face of adversity or trauma. When we eat health-promoting foods, we decrease advanced glycation end products and enrich the body with antioxidants to fight oxidative stress. Antioxidant-rich foods sacrifice themselves against those harmful free radicals, like a bodyguard protecting a celebrity by donating electrons. They stand guard in the body, keeping you from harm's way. And they not only protect you from bad things happening, they promote endothelium health —that highway that can direct you toward heart disease or heart health. Where can we find these free radical inhibiting antioxidants? We find them in fruits, vegetables, whole grains, beans, legumes, nuts, seeds, and spices rich in a multitude of phytonutrients including vitamins and minerals such as beta-carotene, other carotenoids, vitamins A, C, E, and selenium.

Vitamin C can be sourced from foods like oranges, black currants, kiwi, strawberries, broccoli, and spinach. Vitamin E is abundant in avocados, seeds, and whole grains. Selenium, which plays a protective role for the kidneys and prostate, can be found in whole grains and Brazil nuts. Nuts also contain essential minerals like manganese, zinc, and copper. Carotene, a precursor to vitamin A, is present in foods such as pumpkin, mangoes, apricots, and carrots. Spinach, parsley, and kale are rich in vitamins A, C, E, and K. When it comes to nourishing your body, plant-based foods offer an ideal combination of fiber, carbohydrates, proteins, and fats, naturally enriched with the micronutrients necessary to enhance your resilience and ultimately support your overall health.

The Relationship Between Resilient Food and Perceived Stress

The brain is one of the most highly perfused organs in the body, receiving up to 20% of the cardiac output (the blood volume ejected) from the heart with every contraction. This network of vasculature in the brain is lined with endothelial cells similar to what was described for the remainder of the body, so it is not surprising that the foods we eat will impact our brain and therefore our perceived stress. There are a number of studies that look at the impact of eating habits on perceived stress. In one study, the researchers wanted to answer this question: "Is there a relationship between eating fruits and vegetables and stress levels?" They found that people who ate at least two cups of fruits and vegetables daily had 10% lower stress levels than those who consumed less than one cup daily. Another study that looked at a multitude of different studies, a meta-analysis, provided further evidence that fruit and vegetable intake was protective against depression. An additional study showed that eating one and a half ounces of dark chocolate rich in antioxidants during a two-week period reduced perceived stress in females. Most people do not need a study to confirm that chocolate lifts their moods!

There was a study to determine the effectiveness of probiotics on stress. Probiotics occur naturally in the body and in many fermented foods, though yogurt is probably the one we are most familiar with. Less known probiotic foods are kimchi and kombucha. Probiotics subjectively reduce stress levels, and they may raise the threshold at which one feels more anxious and stressed.

Is One Dietary Pattern Really Better For Mood?

You may wonder if one food plan is better than another. Let's defer to the research. A 2012 study took 39 omnivores, or meat-eaters, and divided them into three groups. One group continued to eat meat. Another group ate fish, and the third group ate vegetables. A food frequency questionnaire, a mood questionnaire, and a depression, anxiety, and stress scale questionnaire were taken at the beginning of the study and again after two weeks of consuming the assigned eating parameters. After two weeks, researchers found that the mood scores for the whole food vegetable and fruit consuming participants improved significantly compared to those who ate the omnivore and pescatarian diets.

Australia leads the field on food's impact on mood. So let us address some of the studies from down under. Research published in 2022 looked at over 8,000 Australian adults. They found that a higher consumption of fruits and vegetables were associated with lower odds of worries, tension, and lack of joy. The authors suggested that following dietary guidelines for the recommended intake of fruits and vegetables may ease worries and tensions and make people more joyful. Another Australian study looked at adults equally represented by men and women. The study showed that higher consumption of fruits and vegetables is associated with lower odds of having perceived stress. They recommended eating the rainbow of food colors like apples, pears, oranges, bananas, blueberries, and strawberries along with cruciferous vegetables like broccoli, kale, and bok choy. Other foods in our rainbow of foods include red, orange, and yellow legumes. Eating a wide array of vegetables can assist in preventing or reducing perceived stress. These results align with the outcomes of a significant study in the United States known as the Nurses' Health Study, which showed that consistently eating fruits and vegetables throughout one's lifetime is associated with a reduced likelihood of experiencing depression or sadness as one gets older.

The famed GEICO study, led by the Physicians Committee for Responsible Medicine, determined the effects of fruits and vegetables as they relate to perceived stress. Researchers found that a dietary intervention that moves participants toward a plant-based diet improved depression, anxiety, and productivity in a multicenter corporate setting.

These studies offer evidence that food matters in stress management. What we eat adds to resiliency or stress. What we eat affects our perception of stress. Adopting and embracing the mantra of nutritional resiliency can transform your diet, and a new diet might just be the secret sauce that allows you to thrive rather than flail around in life.

How Fruits and Vegetables Influence Mood

One proposed mechanism for the impact of fruits and vegetables on mood is related to their effects on the gut microbiome. The gut microbiome comprises a community of microorganisms residing in the digestive tract, and it plays a vital role in regulating mood and mental well-being. Fruits and vegetables are rich in fiber, which serves as nourishment for beneficial gut bacteria and supports a healthy microbiome. A balanced gut microbiome has been associated with improved mood and reduced rates of depression and anxiety.

Another proposed mechanism involves the influence of fruits and vegetables on reducing inflammation within the body. Persistent inflammation has been linked to an increased risk of depression and other mood disorders. Fruits and vegetables are abundant sources of antioxidants and other anti-inflammatory compounds, which can help mitigate inflammation and contribute to better mental health.

Nuts and seeds are excellent sources of tryptophan, an amino acid that acts as a precursor to serotonin, a neurotransmitter crucial for mood regulation. Fruits and vegetables have been shown to enhance the conversion of tryptophan into serotonin. Some studies suggest that a diet rich in a combination of nuts, fruits, and vegetables may elevate serotonin levels, potentially leading to improved mood. In summary, the beneficial effects of fruits and vegetables on mood likely result from a combination of factors, encompassing their influence on the gut microbiome, inflammation, neurotransmitter levels, as well as the psychological benefits of embracing a nutritious diet.

Consuming Resilient Foods: Benefits to the Heart and Beyond

It's essential to recognize that eating a whole food, plant-based diet isn't a universal remedy for all health or mental well-being issues; however, it serves as a pivotal element or the core of a Selfish approach. Let's delve into how diet impacts various aspects of the body beyond heart health.

The DASH diet, or "Dietary Approaches to Stop Hypertension," was developed by Dr. Frank Sacks and his team, inspired by the lower blood pressure observed in individuals following a vegetarian diet. This diet aimed to harness the benefits of plant-based foods while accommodating non-vegetarians by allowing some animal product inclusion. Research in the 1990s showed that dietary modifications alone could reduce systolic blood pressure by 6 to 11 points, comparable to standard dosing of many anti-hypertensive medications. Beyond blood pressure, the DASH diet improves blood glucose, triglycerides, and LDL cholesterol, aids in weight management, and supports heart health. It also lowers the risk of colorectal cancer and benefits various health conditions. In contrast to the creators of the DASH diet, the Self*ish* plan advocates for a complete shift toward a whole food, plant-based diet. Partially adopting a whole food, plant-based diet is akin to taking only a fraction of a prescribed medication when it is evident that the full dosage yields the greatest benefits.

Another study encompassing more than one million participants found that incorporating a whole food, plant-based diet into one's eating habits can reduce the risk of cardiovascular disease and cancer mortality. A meta-analysis of 18 cohort studies reinforced these findings, indicating a 9% reduction in the overall risk of death, a 14% decrease in the risk of fatal heart attacks, and a 3% reduction in the risk of cancer-related mortality.

Let's revisit a study I mentioned earlier known as "The Reasons for Geographic and Racial Differences in Stroke," conducted in Alabama. This study goes beyond examining stroke outcomes. Southern-style cuisine, deeply embedded in our culture, isn't necessarily compatible with our bodies. Those tempting fried foods, organ meats, eggs, processed meats, and sugary beverages, while they may appeal to the taste buds of some, they are less than ideal for our health. These investigations have shown that embracing a predominantly whole food, plant-based diet instead of the traditional Southern diet resulted in a 41% lower risk of heart failure, while following a Southern diet increased heart failure risk by 72%. The authors additionally showed that adhering to the whole food, plant-based diet significantly diminishes the risk of heart attacks, sudden cardiac arrest, stroke, Alzheimer's or cognitive impairment, and end-stage kidney disease.

Our food choices wield tremendous power. They impact our well-being across multiple dimensions, influencing not only our physical health but also our stress levels and moods. Additional studies have examined the broader risk of mortality. One study found that substituting just 3% of calories from processed meats with plant proteins can lead to a remarkable 46% reduction in cardiovascular events. Another study indicated that replacing 3% of energy derived from specific animal protein sources with plant protein results in lower mortality rates, particularly when replacing egg protein, resulting in a 15-39% lower risk in men and a 17-34% lower risk in women for overall mortality, cancer, cardiovascular disease, heart disease, and respiratory disease mortality. Similarly, substituting 3% of energy from red meat protein with plant protein led to mortality reductions of 11-25% in both sexes for various causes of mortality. Replacing dairy protein with plant protein was also associated with lower mortality rates in both men and women. These studies demonstrate that even small changes can have profound effects on your health.

The Transformational Power of Plant-Based Foods

In different parts of the world, two important studies, the Mt. Abu Open Heart Trial and the Lifestyle Heart Trial, looked at the effects of including fruits, vegetables, whole grains, and legumes in people's diets. Despite being conducted in different places, both studies found that adding these plant-based foods to a healthy lifestyle could actually reverse the narrowing of arteries, a condition known as atherosclerosis.

While it may seem too good to be true, recent research conducted in 2023 revealed that even minor changes in our lifestyle can make a significant impact on our health. According to the study, a mere 1% reduction in artery plaque could lead to a substantial 25% decrease in serious heart-related problems like heart attacks and death. The results of this research, when combined with the Mt. Abu Open Heart Trial and the Lifestyle Heart Trial, strongly suggest that a diet rich in whole plant foods, fiber, and essential nutrients can play a pivotal role in preventing and potentially reversing heart disease by enhancing blood vessel function, leading to a reduction in atherosclerosis and consequently reducing the risk of heart disease.

Dr. Dean Ornish, lead author in the Lifestyle Heart Trial, led a study on prostate cancer, where he combined a whole food, plant-based diet with stress reduction, quitting smoking, and regular exercise as a therapeutic intervention. Men in this program saw a significant drop in a specific marker for prostate cancer, while those who didn't make these changes saw an increase in the marker. The blood from those following the healthy lifestyle was also more effective at stopping prostate cancer cells from growing. Similar positive results were seen in a study on breast cancer, where a low-fat, high-fiber diet combined with daily exercise reduced risk factors for breast cancer and slowed the growth of cancer cells.

Another study demonstrating the transformational power of plant-based foods focused on colon cancer in African Americans. Researchers swapped the diets of African Americans in Pittsburgh with a group of West Africans. The African Americans, who initially had early-stage colon cancer, started eating a high-fiber, low-fat African-style diet, while the West Africans received a high-fat, low-fiber Western-style diet. Surprisingly, the African Americans' blood profiles improved after changing their diets, while the West Africans who adopted the American diet showed signs of precancerous changes in just two weeks. These findings highlight how our eating habits can affect the risk of colon cancer and how adopting healthier diets can reverse markers associated with cancer development.

In essence, our DNA is not our Destiny. Our dietary choices hold significant sway over our health, affecting various facets of our well-being, from physical health to stress levels and emotional states.

How Fruits and Vegetables Heal a Heart

Fruits and vegetables offer a cornucopia of nutrients and bioactive compounds that bestow significant advantages to heart health. Here are some key ways in which fruits and vegetables can wield their beneficial influence on the heart:

Nitric Oxide (NO) Production: Nitric oxide stands as a pivotal molecule, meticulously crafted by endothelial cells, and is indispensable for the regulation of blood flow and blood pressure. Vegetables serve as rich reservoirs of nitrates, which undergo transformation into NO within our bodies. Research has compellingly shown that the ingestion of nitrates from foods such as beets and leafy greens can amplify NO production, ultimately bolstering endothelial function.

Antioxidants: Abundantly graced with antioxidants, fruits and vegetables play a crucial role in diminishing oxidative stress within the body. Oxidative stress can inflict damage upon endothelial cells, impairing their proper function. Antioxidants act as vigilant sentinels, shielding these cells from harm and fostering enhanced endothelial function.

Polyphenols: Fruits and vegetables also teem with polyphenols, bioactive compounds renowned for their prowess in boosting endothelial function. Polyphenols have been scientifically acknowledged for their role in stimulating NO production, mitigating inflammation, and ameliorating vascular tone.

Fiber: A vital nutrient exclusively found in plant-based foods, fiber plays a significant role in elevating endothelial function. Fiber aids in quelling inflammation within the body and nurtures a healthier gut microbiome, which in turn supports endothelial function. Fiber also exerts a substantial influence on cholesterol levels.

Fiber engages in a binding dance with bile acids in the intestine, facilitating their removal from the body. Since bile acids originate from cholesterol, their elimination prods the liver to utilize more cholesterol to produce fresh bile acids, thereby contributing to reduced overall cholesterol levels.

Moreover, fiber acts as a gatekeeper, slowing down the absorption of cholesterol within the intestine, preventing it from entering the bloodstream. Soluble fiber, in particular, exhibits remarkable prowess in lowering cholesterol levels. Foods such as oats, barley, legumes, and select fruits and vegetables stand as rich reservoirs of soluble fiber. While the recommended daily intake of fiber is 25 grams for women and 38 grams for men, many individuals fall short of these guidelines. Upping the consumption of high-fiber foods, including whole grains, fruits, vegetables, and legumes, can substantially lower cholesterol levels and reduce the risk of heart disease.

Fiber Facilitates Weight Loss: The consumption of high-fiber foods fosters a heightened sense of fullness and contentment, contributing to a reduction in overall calorie intake and bolstering weight loss endeavors. This effect is orchestrated through various mechanisms. Soluble fiber, in particular, plays a pivotal role in regulating hormones linked to appetite control. Multiple studies have affirmed that soluble fiber intake reduces the production of hunger-inducing hormones, such as ghrelin, while simultaneously stimulating the production of satiety-promoting hormones like cholecystokinin, GLP-1, and peptide YY. Notably, the weight loss medication Ozempic capitalizes on the GLP-1 pathway. Additionally, fiber curtails appetite by decelerating the transit of food through the digestive tract. The gradual release of nutrients like glucose into the gut prompts a more gradual insulin response, which, in turn, dampens the sensation of hunger. Weight loss can be instrumental in lowering cholesterol levels, especially the notorious LDL cholesterol.

Fiber and Gut Health: Fiber promotes the flourishing of beneficial gut bacteria, an influence that can positively impact overall health and metabolism. Some studies have hinted at a correlation between the gut microbiome, cholesterol metabolism, and the development of heart disease.

The Healing

I understood Angie more than she realized. I had my own healing journey, and it was a journey filled with study, research, and countless "ah-ha"s. I remember how proud my dad was when I finished medical school. He wanted to be a doctor, but circumstances blocked his path. His dad died when he was 13. Later he moved from Louisiana to California and lived with his older brother. He fought and scratched his way to achieve success. His optimistic, hopeful personality never allowed him to stop; when he encountered an obstacle, he would trailblaze other pathways. He forged on as an educator and businessman, always burning the midnight oil to ensure his family had all we needed in life. He expected success; he encouraged success. Dad birthed success into existence. Then there was this great exception because when it came to his health, he malfunctioned. I don't remember a time when my dad did not use insulin to treat his diabetes. I shouldn't have been surprised that after attending four years of medical school, three years of internal medicine, three years of general cardiology, and one year of interventional cardiology, my father's life had drastically changed. I had been absorbed for 11 years with my medical education. When I finally came up for air and began spending more time with my father, he was no longer the strong figure I knew when I was younger. While I was learning how to help people, diabetes waged a silent war in my dad's body. It is said we are in a constant silent battle pitting wellness vs illness, and diabetes was winning. It damaged his eyes, leaving him legally blind. It ravaged his nervous system, leaving his foot without feeling and the inability to flex his foot. He begrudgingly used a walker to safely move around, and to top everything off, he could no longer drive. He had to wait for my mom to take him places or find another way. When I looked at him as an adult, I saw a man who was now only a shell of his former self.

I'm not sure if it was guilt or just a desire to give my dad a little joy, but I decided to buy him a special pair of dress shoes. He needed custom shoes to fit the leg brace that was needed to keep his foot from dropping as a result of the nerve damage in his foot. My dad loved to dress up. He frequently wore business suits and presented himself in the utmost professional way. He always had a pair of dress shoes. I emulated my dad's dress code. As a youngster, I shined my shoes so that I could walk outside looking polished like my dad. It troubled my dad that he could no longer wear nice shoes because of the braces. I thought these special shoes would be a treat for him. I found a company that made dress shoes that could accommodate his braces. When I took him to look at the different shoe styles, he lit up with childlike pleasure. He told me that he was starting to feel like himself again. His pleasure brought joy into both our lives that day. As I mentioned, diabetes damages the nerves, and that not only causes the foot to drop but it also prevents patients from feeling their feet or feeling pain. The shoes I bought my dad produced pressure on his foot that he couldn't feel, and that pressure eventually led to a blister. The blister led to an ulceration that got infected. In time, this condition rendered him unable to walk.

Over the next year or two, my dad's health continued to spiral down. Once when I'd planned to go out of town, I stopped by to see my father before I left. When I walked in to see him, he was in bed, and I saw that look on his face that I'd seen many times before in patients who were nearing death. I knew my dad didn't have long on this earth. I was torn up on the inside, knowing that my wonderful dad was leaving. That day, without anyone telling them to come, all my brothers and sisters visited. It was divine intervention. It was a reflection of who my dad was as a person. The support he received during his last hours was extremely important, not just for him but for all the family, and dad received what he needed. That day, my dad died, and my heart thrashed in my chest. It was the day my life changed forever, and not just because of his death. After all, I was grown and could take care of myself. It was something else. I was living a life built on his back, and I'd failed him. I felt guilty. I felt responsible, and as I related earlier in the book, I wondered if there was something I could have done to prevent his decline and death.

Those were dark times. As I relate the story, I can still feel my guts churn. I moved in slow motion for weeks after the funeral services. I felt like a fraud when a patient thanked me for helping them. Every time I heard "thank you," the internal voice of guilt shouted at me. This is where the seeds of resiliency, planted by my amazing parents, began to flourish. Just like dad, who never allowed life to steamroll him, I would not let life, guilt, or the past take me down. It was better to honor my father's legacy by fully living than to limp along immobilized by circumstances. Again, I was flooded with gratitude for all the lessons that allowed me to handle life's ups and downs, especially the downs. As I said earlier, I tried to recall my dad's medical history. What was missing? I became an investigative journalist. I felt like I was stumbling in the dark until I found the book *Prevent and Reverse Heart Disease* by Dr. Caldwell Esselstyn, whom I now call my mentor. It was the chapter called Moderation Kills that stopped me in my tracks. I related the words to my father's journey. He didn't smoke. He didn't drink. He didn't do drugs. Of course, he ate, but by society's standards he ate moderately. But his diet was harmful enough to feed the simmering flames of inflammation. When the inflammation levels are low and even moderate, they become undetectable by traditional tests. That means that the destruction done to the body flies under the radar. And to be clear, this means there is ongoing damage occurring in the body, even when the person is asymptomatic or the damage is undetectable. Just because we can't measure it doesn't mean it's not there. This situation is akin to prescribing medications. I could give one patient a lower dosage and they might have a bad reaction immediately. It was clear that they could not tolerate the medicine. With other patients, they could take higher and higher doses before they had a bad reaction. It's the same with food. Some people can tolerate a lifetime of poor eating habits and not have any perceivable adverse outcomes while others will have bad reactions after eating poorly for a short period of time. The problem is that food is everywhere. Food is culture. Food is who we are. The drawback is that we don't know how the food we eat will affect us until it's too late!

I drank in the research as if I were dying of thirst. My mind did double flips, and I felt as if I was solving the mystery behind illness and disease. The research was so compelling that I changed my lifestyle. After all, good nutrition had the power to heal and transform my health. I became a cheerleader for better eating, better health, but my newfound zeal did not land well with everyone. Some friends and family members looked at me as if I had lost it. "What is he doing now? Why is he always trying something different?" They did not understand. As I said, food is culture, and going against cultural norms is not always easy. I felt guilty because I had to forgo certain long-term eating rituals with people I cared about. There were restaurants I would no longer frequent. I felt like I was breaking an invisible code of loyalty, but I persisted. It took a lot of grit, but I could not ignore the gripping evidence. I persevered in adopting a whole food, plant-based diet. I had more energy, and though this may seem like a stretch to believe, I began to heal emotionally. I'm not sure if it was because I was thinking more clearly or if it was somehow just helping to heal those wounds that had surfaced after my dad died.

I mentioned the dark times immediately after my dad died. It was during that period when I was sleepwalking through life. I didn't pay attention to the simple things in life, and I even allowed my life insurance to lapse. As I regained my focus and clarity on life, I needed to get my life insurance reinstated. I met with my financial planner, and she worked it out so I could get reinstated. This involved getting a physical and having my bloodwork done. I was a bit nervous about the tests. It had been five years since the last insurance physical. At that time, I was designated as a preferred risk. Now I was five years older. I was amazed when I received the results. I came back labeled super preferred! Here's the back story. I had told my financial planner I wanted to repeat the tests. I planned to fast and work out more. I was rigorous in implementing the Self*ish* plan and then I was retested. When the results came back, my financial planner said, "Columbus, do you realize that nobody moves from preferred to super preferred, especially when they are five years older. I'm not sure what you've been doing, but whatever it is, keep doing it!"

At this point in my life, I had to change the way I conducted my practice. The research told me that some things must change. Though my medical training provided the bricks in my practice, it was the books I read, the research I studied, and my personal health results that provided the mortar. And you can't build a solid structure without both bricks and mortar. It was as if there was a reckoning in my life, and I thought of this new path, this new way, as a kind of penance for my ignorance, my lack of knowledge, and my lack of understanding despite being medically trained. It was my training, or lack of the right kind of training, that led to my inability to help my dad. I wanted to make amends by sharing this information with a wide audience. As you can see from my story about Angie, I started with my patients. I lovingly encouraged them to read certain books while I developed a structure to help with lifestyle changes. This structure ultimately became the Self*ish*-program. Once my patients read the literature, I helped them institute lifestyle changes. I realized the department of cardiology desperately needed to integrate nutrition into its arsenal of therapeutic interventions, so I hired a dietitian. I created the Integrative Cardiovascular Disease Program, where I hosted in-house patient-focused lectures. The lectures eventually evolved into cooking sessions. I offered services that provided my patients with the "why" they needed to make changes and how to make these changes. I called these cooking sessions the CATH lab, an acronym for cooking alternatives to health. I chose this name with forethought because a cath lab is also the place where cardiologists perform heart procedures. This is where we try to prevent or stop a heart attack and where procedures transform symptoms. This is where the magic happens, allowing people to get a second chance at life. And that's what I was doing with the cooking sessions. I was providing people with a second chance. It was another sort of cath lab. If someone adopted the principles I taught in these sessions, they could have a second chance at life. They could put their disease in remission. They could extend their lives if they would adopt whole food, plant-based eating.

Since I incorporated lifestyle into my practice of cardiology and interventional cardiology, I've been blessed to witness patients in different age groups, backgrounds, ethnicities, and genders heal. Like a proud father, I watched their symptoms resolve, their heart function improve, and their relationships heal.

When I shared this story with Angie, I told her that she could break the cycle of food addiction. She could heal emotionally. "I know this, Angie, because I've experienced it myself. It is possible. There is power in these choices, and you have the ability to restore your mind and your body. You have the power to choose what you eat and the power to take care of yourself."

In the movie *Castaway*, Tom Hanks portrayed a character who was stranded on a deserted island and found solace in a volleyball named Wilson, which he personified as his sole companion and source of support. While this served as a coping mechanism during his difficult times, it's important to note that the movie didn't conclude with his reliance on this fake resource. In fact, he eventually escaped the island with Wilson on a raft, but in a gripping scene, Wilson bounced off the raft and drifted beyond his reach. This forced Tom's character to make a heart-wrenching decision between saving Wilson or his own life on the raft. He ultimately chose to let go of Wilson and swim back to the raft, recognizing that it was the only way to save himself.

If you're reading this and can relate to Tom's character, it's possible that you too have relied on a fake resource to cope with stress in an effort to heal your broken heart. However, it's important to realize that in order to truly heal, you may need to let go of this fake resource. It will require you to get Sel*fish* and have a willingness to prioritize your own health and well-being. But know that you're capable of making this difficult choice and achieving the healing you deserve.

I hope I have convinced you of the importance of food choices and what you eat in regard to your health. I cannot emphasize enough the urgency of making healthy food choices. Start small. Make healthier food choices, and transition into eating healthier and healthier foods. This chapter provides vital information for your heart health and for your overall health. Use it as a guide and a motivational source in transitioning to a better lifestyle. And as the old saying goes, you are what you eat.

Can I just take a supplement?

Angie's question was a common one that came up whenever I began to describe getting Sel*fish* with one's diet to heal a broken heart. Fifty-two percent of the U.S. population is taking supplements, and it's big business, with Americans spending over 30 billion dollars annually on dietary supplements. Such rampant use of supplements raises the question: Should I take a supplement? Randomized controlled trials have generally failed to show significant benefits of commonly used supplements such as multivitamins, vitamin D, calcium, and vitamin C for CVD or all-cause mortality. However, folic acid, B vitamins, and selenium may have potential benefits. Folic acid has been shown to reduce stroke and total CVD in China, where there is no folic acid food fortification, while B-complex mixtures of folic acid, B12, and B6 have been used to treat high homocysteine levels associated with stroke. Slow-release niacin has been found to increase all-cause mortality with no CVD advantage and may cause liver damage and worsen diabetes control. Finally, when selenium is included in an antioxidant mixture, there are possible benefits for CVD and all-cause mortality.

Red Yeast Rice

Red yeast rice can mildly reduce cholesterol, triglycerides, and increase HDL cholesterol, as shown in various studies. However, its effectiveness in reducing cardiovascular disease is limited to one large study on Chinese people. For healthy people with mild hypercholesterolemia, low doses of certified citrinin-free Red Yeast Rice with monacolin K can be an effective and safe lipid-lowering nutraceutical. Red Rice Yeast can also be used to enhance the efficacy of other lipid-lowering supplements and non-statin drugs. But it should not replace statins or other LDL-C lowering drugs in high-risk CV patients. Red Rice Yeast extracts with high monacolin K content can cause statin-like adverse events in frail patients and should be used with caution.

Omega 3 Supplementation

Omega-3 PUFAs have many benefits on the cardiovascular system, including improving vascular and endothelial function and reducing inflammation, thrombosis, and plaque composition. They work through various molecular mechanisms. Recent studies using Icosapent Ethyl (IPE), type of omega 3 fatty acid have shown a decrease in ASCVD risk. However, clinical trial data related to omega-3 PUFA supplementation is inconsistent, and more research is needed to determine their clinical indications, effective dose, and formulation. It is recommended to consume food sources of omega-3 PUFAs as part of a heart-healthy diet: flaxseed oil, chia seeds, hemp seeds, walnuts, soybeans and soy products such as tofu and tempeh, leafy green vegetables such as spinach and kale, seaweed and algae-derived supplements (e.g., spirulina, chlorella).

CoQ10

CoQ10 is a common nutritional supplement that plays a major role in helping cells produce energy. It has been studied extensively in humans and animals and is used to help treat two types of heart conditions: statin-associated muscle symptoms (SAMS) and heart failure (HF). These conditions can cause muscle depletion of CoQ10 due to statin medications that can affect the body's ability to make it. The depletion can lead to skeletal muscle pain or heart muscle dysfunction, and CoQ10 supplementation may help. Although CoQ10 is not yet approved by the FDA for treating any medical condition, many doctors still use it to help treat SAMS and HF. More research is needed to fully understand its potential benefits for these conditions, and doctors should continue to explore how it may help patients.

Vitamin D

Low levels of vitamin D have been associated with an elevated risk of cardiovascular disease, yet vitamin D supplements have not demonstrated cardiovascular benefits in studies. Some experts hypothesize that vitamin D levels serve as a proxy for sunlight exposure, explaining why supplementation hasn't shown heart health advantages. This is attributed to the process by which UVB rays from sunlight penetrate the skin, activating endothelial nitric oxide synthase (eNOS) in deeper skin layers, resulting in the production of nitric oxide that relaxes blood vessels, enhancing blood flow and reducing blood pressure. Maintaining a balance is crucial, as excessive sun exposure can lead to sunburn and skin cancer risk. Hence, safeguarding against excessive UV radiation through sunscreen, protective clothing, and sunglasses, particularly during peak sun hours, is vital to mitigate harm while harnessing the benefits of nitric oxide production in the skin.

Some studies suggest that calcium supplements may have potential cardiovascular risks, so they should be used with caution, and people should aim to get their recommended calcium intake from food sources. Plant-based sources for calcium and vitamin D include: leafy green vegetables such as kale, collard greens, and spinach, plant-based milks, such as soy milk or almond milk, tofu made with calcium sulfate, beans and lentils, almonds and other nuts.

L-Arginine

There is some evidence to suggest that oral L-arginine may improve blood flow in certain populations, such as those with peripheral arterial disease or coronary artery disease. This is because L-arginine is a precursor for nitric oxide, which is a molecule that helps to dilate blood vessels and improve blood flow. However, the evidence on the efficacy of L-arginine supplementation for improving blood flow in the general population is mixed, and more research is needed to establish its effects. In one meta-analysis, researchers reviewed 13 studies to see if it really works. They found that taking L-arginine supplements didn't improve blood flow or other measures compared to taking a placebo. So, they concluded that there isn't enough evidence to recommend L-arginine supplements for these conditions.

Transitioning to a Whole Food, Plant-Based Diet

Angie initially grappled with concerns about losing her cultural identity when considering a switch to a whole food, plant-based diet. She understood that food is an integral part of culture, carrying with it traditions, flavors, and stories that connect generations. However, what Angie soon discovered was the beauty of plant-based eating—namely, that every culture across the globe has a rich foundation in plant-centric foods. Drawing from my own family roots in New Orleans, I shared how I grew up watching my mother and grandmother prepare time-tested classics like gumbo, stewed okra, red beans, and collard greens, but with one adjustment—they were completely plant-based. These dishes retained all the flavors and essence of the region they hailed from while emphasizing the abundant plant-based ingredients available. This journey taught Angie that it's not only possible but also enriching to celebrate culturally relevant foods while embracing a plant-focused lifestyle, showing that traditions can thrive without sacrificing health or ethical choices.

As we embark on the journey toward a whole food, plant-based diet, I will guide you through a SMART (Specific, Measurable, Achievable, Relevant, Time-Based) approach to help make a smooth transition to this beneficial way of eating. By setting clear goals and adopting practical strategies, you'll be on your way to enjoying the numerous health benefits of a plant-based lifestyle.

1. **Specify Your Plan:** The first step in adopting a whole food, plant-based diet is to be specific about your goals. Determine what you want to achieve and why it's essential to you. For instance, your goal might be to improve your heart health, lower cholesterol, or increase your energy levels.

2. **Set Measurable Objectives:** Make your goals measurable. Instead of saying you want to "eat more plant-based foods," specify that you aim to "consume at least one cup of fruits and vegetables daily" or "replace one meat-based meal with a plant-based meal each day."

3. **Achievable Changes:** Start with changes that are achievable for you. If you're new to plant-based eating, committing to a 100% plant-based diet from the outset might be challenging. Begin with smaller, attainable steps, like designating certain days of the week as plant-based or opting for plant-based snacks.

4. **Relevance to Your Lifestyle:** Ensure that your goals align with your life and values. A relevant goal is one that makes sense in the context of your daily routine and long-term health. If you have specific dietary preferences or restrictions, tailor your plant-based choices accordingly.

5. **Time-Based Commitment:** Set a specific window of time during which you'll eat plant-based meals. For example, you could decide to have a plant-based breakfast every day for the next two weeks. A time-based commitment helps create structure and accountability.

6. **Focus on What You Add:** Instead of fixating on what you're eliminating, concentrate on what you're adding to your diet. Fill your plate with vibrant, nutrient-rich whole foods like fruits, vegetables, whole grains, legumes, nuts, and seeds. This approach ensures you're nourishing your body while gradually reducing less healthy options.

7. **Eliminate Temptations:** Clear your kitchen of tempting items that don't align with your plant-based goals. Donate or discard processed foods, sugary snacks, and animal products that may undermine your efforts.

8. **Stay Satisfied:** Never let yourself go hungry. Plan your meals and snacks to avoid reaching a state of extreme hunger, which can lead to impulsive, less healthy choices. Keep wholesome plant-based snacks readily available.

9. **Hydration Matters:** Increase your consumption of water. Staying well hydrated is crucial for overall health and can help curb unnecessary cravings. Consider herbal teas, infused water, and hydrating fruits and vegetables like cucumbers and watermelon.

10. **Plan and Record:** Put pen to paper and create a meal plan. Outline your plant-based meals for the week, including breakfast, lunch, dinner, and snacks. Having a plan simplifies grocery shopping and meal preparation.

11. **Bowl Method:** Adopt the bowl method as a practical way to structure your meals. Start with a base of whole grains or colorful starchy vegetables like brown or black rice, or purple potatoes. Add a protein source, such as beans, tofu, or tempeh. Pile on a variety of vegetables like broccoli, kale, collard greens,

or a salad mix. Finish with a flavorful sauce or toppings of your choice.

Remember, transitioning to a whole-food, plant-based diet is a gradual process, and it's okay to progress at your own pace. For additional tips on incorporating a plant based diet into your routine to alleviate stress and foster emotional healing, connect with our community at www.DrBatiste.com.

CHAPTER 6

Intimacy

T he pandemic was a double-edged sword for Angie. Like everyone else, she was forced into social isolation, but her situation became even more heartbreaking when her mother fell ill and was hospitalized. It was a terrible situation - no friends or family were allowed to visit, and her mother rarely saw the overworked doctors and nurses. There were no hugs, no hand-holding, no comforting presence. Angie could only see her mother through video calls, and her mother passed away alone and isolated in the hospital. Learning of her mother's death was devastating for Angie. She felt immense sorrow for not being able to be with her in person and was deeply troubled by the fact that her mother died without the comfort of family by her side. Due to citywide restrictions, the family couldn't even hold a funeral, leaving Angie without closure. For Angie, the pandemic was filled with loss, isolation, and grief, which took a toll on her relationships, particularly her marriage. Her marriage teetered on the edge and eventually crumbled. The combination of stress, isolation, and her mother's lonely death all contributed to her eventual divorce. Angie found herself alone and isolated, but she wasn't the only one facing these challenges. With the declaration of the COVID-19 pandemic by the World Health Organization on March 11, 2020, the world witnessed the closure of businesses and the enforcement of restrictions worldwide, putting life on hold. This sudden change mirrored the lives of approximately 6% of older American adults who live in social isolation and loneliness. As the pandemic continued and a second wave of COVID hit, more closures and restrictions followed, spreading fear and uncertainty across the globe.

In 2023, Dr. Vivek Murthy, the U.S. Surgeon General, declared loneliness as a public health crisis. Research indicates that the beginning of the COVID pandemic led to a 36% increase in loneliness as compared to pre-pandemic surveys, which revealed that 60% of Americans struggle with loneliness. Moreover, 41% of U.S. adults and 58% of adults aged 18-29 experienced high levels of psychological distress at least once during the pandemic. In an effort to determine whether the pandemic caused elevated levels of loneliness, researchers analyzed 34 studies across four continents, mainly focusing on North America and Europe. These long-term studies evaluated the loneliness levels of over 200,000 participants before and during the pandemic. The analysis revealed a modest but noteworthy increase in loneliness during the pandemic. On average, the prevalence of loneliness increased by about 5% across the individual studies. The pandemic caused physical isolation , affecting many individuals, but studies have also confirmed that the pandemic caused emotional stress, leading to loneliness in many individuals. CNBC reported that divorce rates during the pandemic increased. The UK's largest family law firm reported a 95% increase in divorce during the pandemic. Legal Templates reported a 34% increase in divorce agreement contract sales during the first half of 2020, when the lockdown kicked in, compared to the same period in 2018. Subsequent studies called into question the degree of divorces occurring during the pandemic, but there is no doubt that social isolation and loneliness increased exponentially during the pandemic, and relationships across the world eroded.

Intimacy

Webster's Dictionary describes intimacy as a close familiarity or friendship. Intimacy can be emotional or physical and oftentimes both. Emotional intimacy refers to a feeling of closeness with another person. This can be with a sexual partner, but it can also be with close friends or family members. Often, intimate relationships are independent, trusting, and committed. You can rely on those you are intimate with. These people are your tribe, your community. Physical intimacy consists of two people who easily share each other's space. This closeness might occur through a platonic hug or handshake, but it's frequently expressed through more sensual touches like kissing and intercourse. There are innumerable connections between mental well-being and intimacy. Physical and emotional intimacy can impact and be impacted by mental health. Intimate interpersonal relationships make up a large component of mental health. Close relationships give you a strong support system, which is invaluable during an illness. Intimacy helps fight symptoms of certain mental health disorders. During 2020, we saw a global experiment that revealed the impact of isolation and loss of intimacy.

Loneliness

Loneliness is undoubtedly the opposite of intimacy. Though loneliness and social isolation differ, they are closely related. Loneliness is the distressing feeling of being alone or separated while social isolation is the lack of social contacts. People can live alone and not feel lonely, while others can be in a crowd and feel lonely. I didn't understand this until after my dad passed away. Mom could be surrounded by family or friends and later she might remark that she felt lonely. She had friends and family, but to her, it was not the same. Nothing was ever the same after my dad passed. Mom suffered a tremendous loss. Her relationship with her children differed from her relationship with her husband. She missed his familiar touch and the intimacy they shared. Loneliness can be defined as the distress that results from discrepancies between the ideal and perceived social relationships. The keyword here is "perceived." Loneliness is not the same experience as that of being alone. If you perceive that your relationship should be more engaging or different, you may feel negatively impacted. This perception causes a sense of distress, and this sense of lack leads to a cascade of bodily events that impact our health and well-being.

The Biology of Intimacy

The biology of intimacy involves various physiological and neurochemical processes that occur in the brain and body when humans form close emotional connections with others. Intimacy, which can refer to emotional closeness, social bonding, and attachment, is a fundamental aspect of human relationships and can have significant biological implications. Most scientists probably have experienced intimacy, but being scientists, they wanted to see what happens in the brain when we experience intimacy or the lack of intimacy. They discovered that when mice are isolated for 24 hours, they tend to crave the company of other mice. The mechanism that facilitates this craving is shown through a brain scan. Brain images reveal that the dorsal raphe nuclei (The dorsal raphe nucleus is like a factory in your brain that helps you feel good and balanced. It's an essential part of your brain's control center, making sure your emotions and mood stay on track.), which is sensitive to social isolation, activates and releases dopamine. The dopamine does its work, then recedes. We remember that dopamine is a messenger hormone that motivates us to act. It may drive us toward a particular pleasure-seeking activity or toward an emotionally healing activity. The dopamine release corresponds with this craving or this drive toward being in social contact. The research took into account visual activation, since it can trigger a state of loneliness. Researchers found that when there was enough social contact, dopamine release was inhibited.

The Biology of Loneliness

Loneliness is the distress that results from discrepancies between ideal and perceived relationships; therefore, loneliness is a type of perceived psychological stress that induces and triggers stress hormones. Studies demonstrate that loneliness activates the fight or flight response. I remember after my dad died, while visiting my mom, she would describe individuals or cars parked near her home at very odd hours. Her loneliness had created a hyper-vigilance that kept her from sleeping and imprisoned her in a fight-or-flight mindset. Loneliness has also been shown to activate the immune system. This leads to increased activation of white blood cells, which in turn increases inflammation. While inflammation is a natural response to a wound or a bacterial infection, when these chemicals cannot be used in a natural way, they serve as triggers to many diseases, including atherosclerosis, or hardening of the vessels. Researchers looked at lonely people and monkeys who were socially isolated and found that they had more inflammation and less effective immune responses compared to those who were not lonely. Loneliness also affected how certain genes were expressed in their immune cells. The study showed that loneliness can lead to the production of immature immune cells that are more likely to cause inflammation in the body. This can make it harder for the body to fight off viruses and other infections. The study suggested that loneliness can create a cycle where it leads to more health problems, and these health problems can make people feel even more lonely.

Impact of Loneliness on Overeating

In order to further understand the biology of loneliness, scientists did a study to learn about how feeling lonely might make people eat too much. They used a special machine called functional magnetic resonance imaging (fMRI) to look at people's brains. They asked 40 adult volunteers to do two 10-hour activities: one where they couldn't eat food, and another where they couldn't talk to anyone, not even a friend or family member. They took pictures of the volunteers' brains right after each activity. While in the machine, the volunteers saw pictures of things they liked, such as their favorite foods or ways of being with others, like hanging out with friends. They also saw pictures of flowers as a comparison. The scientists found that a certain part of the brain reacted to the pictures based on what the volunteers had been deprived of, like food or social contact, and how hungry or lonely they felt. It was interesting that the brain reacted similarly when the volunteers were fasting or feeling lonely. This suggests that feeling lonely might make our brains crave food, just like when we're hungry. This helps explain why some people gained more weight, up to 27%, during the early stages of the pandemic when they were socially disconnected. We want to be close to others so much that when we feel lonely, our brains might make us try to fill that void with something else, like food.

The Impact of Loneliness on Health

In 2017, former US surgeon General Vivek Murthy drew awareness to loneliness when he called it an epidemic. Researchers find that the odds of mortality or death due to social isolation and loneliness are similar to someone smoking up to 15 cigarettes per day and drinking 6 alcoholic drinks per day. This risk caused by loneliness is higher than the risks posed by physical inactivity and obesity, which are major contributors to chronic disease and death. Other population-based studies, which means looking at individuals across the United States or the world, have demonstrated that both social isolation and the perception of social isolation or loneliness are related to a higher risk of mortality. And social isolation and loneliness are risk factors for a broken heart. In 2022, a study published in American Heart Association assessed 44,000 postmenopausal women from the Women's Health Initiative study and found that socially isolated women had a higher risk of developing heart failure (HF), even after accounting for other risk factors.

Depressive symptoms did not mediate this association, and age and race/ethnicity did not moderate it. The study suggests that social isolation is independently associated with increased risk of HF in older women. A 2023 study published in the *Journal American College of Cardiology* identified similar results, but this time evaluating over 460,000 individuals. They found that both social isolation and loneliness were associated with a higher likelihood of developing heart failure, even after accounting for genetic risk. Interestingly, the association between social isolation and heart failure risk was influenced by loneliness status. Other studies have shown that lonely people have elevated blood pressure. Even socially isolated animals are more inclined to have atherosclerosis, endothelial damage, or a reduction in vessel dilation.

Grief, Loneliness and Depression

Approximately 35% of adults aged 45 years and older, and over 40% of adults aged 60 years and older, report feeling lonely, with more than one in five experiencing severe loneliness. The loss of a loved one can intensify feelings of loneliness in older adults. For example, bereaved individuals often report feeling lonely, with 70% of older widows and widowers describing loneliness as the most challenging aspect to cope with on a daily basis. Loneliness has also been found to be a gateway to developing depressive symptoms in some bereaved individuals. One example of the connection between grief, loneliness, and depression is the life of former President Calvin Coolidge.

In the book *The Tormented President: Calvin Coolidge, Death, and Clinical Depression* by Robert E. Gilbert, it is argued that Calvin Coolidge, the 30th president of the United States, stopped functioning effectively as president after the death of his 16-year-old son, Calvin Jr. The book describes how Calvin Jr. died from an infection caused by a blister on his toe, and how Coolidge was deeply affected by this loss, as well as by earlier losses in his life, including the death of his mother when he was twelve and his younger sister five years later. Coolidge exhibited symptoms of major depression, including loss of appetite, insomnia, agitation, decreased energy, and recurrent thoughts of death, among others. After Calvin Jr.'s death, Coolidge became less engaged in his presidential duties, slept more, and delegated more responsibilities to his wife, cabinet, and congress. He also became less communicative with the press, earning the nickname "Silent Cal." Four years after leaving the presidency, Calvin Coolidge died suddenly of a heart attack. Since his death in 1933, researchers have identified a relationship between depression and heart attacks.

In 2017, research by the National Heart, Lung, and Blood Institute showed that adults with depressive symptoms or a depressive disorder have a 64% greater risk of developing CAD than the general population, and CAD patients with depression are 59% more likely to have a future adverse cardiovascular event. One proposed cause of the relationship between grief/loneliness/depression and heart attacks is increased activity of platelets. Platelets are tiny cells in our blood that help our body stop bleeding when we get hurt. They are like little superheroes that rush to the site of an injury to form a plug and stop the bleeding. However, sometimes platelets can also cause problems in our heart. When we have a heart attack, it usually happens because our blood vessels leading to the heart are blocked. This blockage can be caused by a buildup of fatty substances in the blood vessels called plaques. When a plaque ruptures or breaks open, it can trigger our platelets to form a clot around the rupture site. This clot can get bigger and completely block the blood vessel, preventing blood flow to the heart. This is bad because our heart needs blood and oxygen to function properly.

Scientists have discovered that platelets could be a missing link between heart disease, chronic stress, and depressive symptoms. In a study published in the *Journal of Neuroimmune Pharmacology*, researchers looked at how acute (short-term) and chronic (long-term) mental stress affected platelet activity in healthy male participants.

They found that chronic mental stress, which could be caused by things like grief or loneliness, led to increased feelings of anxiety, depressive symptoms, and perceived stress. Platelets from participants with chronic stress showed increased markers of inflammation and activation. Acute mental stress, which could be caused by things like exams or public speaking, also caused changes in platelet activity, including increased activation markers and platelet-leukocyte aggregates, which are clumps of platelets and other cells stuck together. The ability of platelets to recover from acute stress was impaired by chronic stress, meaning that the platelets did not return to normal as quickly. This suggests that mental stress can cause increased and prolonged inflammation in platelets, which could help explain the link between mental health and physical health disorders.

In simpler terms, platelets are not only important in stopping bleeding but they may also be involved in our body's response to stress. When we experience stress, especially for a long time, it can affect our platelets and cause them to become more active and inflamed. This could be one of the reasons why stress is linked to both mental health and physical health problems, like heart disease.

Does Being Single Increase My Risk of Heart Disease?

It would seem that being single could easily play a role in developing heart disease due to the stressful effects of being lonely or from social isolation. That's not the case. Being single does not automatically mean that a single person is lonely or socially isolated. A single person may have a large social community. They may have deep, sustaining friendships and support systems. They may perceive that their interactions and bonds are strong enough to support them through good and bad times.

What happens when a single person has no confidante? No one they trust, or no one to count on? A 1992 study revealed that coronary heart disease patients who were not married and did not have a confidante had a significantly higher five-year risk of dying. Their risk of dying was 50% compared to the 18% observed in the patients with a spouse or partner. The study did not address whether the spouse's or partner's relationship was healthy or toxic, but they did infer that someone who had a confidante enjoyed better health benefits. A Harvard-based study of adult development found that stable relationships that were developed by a person's midlife are better predictors of being healthy and happy 30 years later than cholesterol levels. This demonstrates once again the power of relationships.

Loneliness and Hypertension in Cardiovascular Disease

I've already described a set of occurrences that lead to disease states like elevated blood pressure. Large-scale studies show that there is an association between increased blood pressure and loneliness, especially as we age. One of the key factors is that our social connections decrease as we get older, and the fewer social ties, the higher our blood pressure is likely to be. This has been confirmed repeatedly by multiple study reviews: Loneliness is related to elevated blood pressure and other stress markers. It's no surprise that there is a relationship with loneliness as a stressor leading to issues like Broken Heart Syndrome and coronary heart disease. A meta-analysis that reviewed multiple trials reported a 29% higher risk for initial heart disease and stroke in individuals with high versus low levels of loneliness or social isolation.

A 2022 study report in the *Journal of American Medical Association* revealed that both social isolation and loneliness were independently associated with a higher risk of cardiovascular disease in post-menopausal women—women like Angie. Women with both social isolation and loneliness have greater cardiovascular risks than those with either exposure alone. Think about that; let it sink in. When we are isolated and we have fewer connections to others, the risk of developing some form of cardiovascular disease is exponentially higher. A Swedish study with more than 17,000 participants found that those with the fewest social contacts were at a 50% higher risk of dying of cardiovascular disease. But here's the silver lining: When a woman has a heart problem, having friends actually can improve her chances of survival. Another study found that women with suspected coronary artery disease were more than twice as likely to be alive after two years if they had a wide social circle. What's more, they had lower rates of hypertension and diabetes. I hope these statistics convince you of the importance of having friends and community. These connections are literally lifesaving.

American Heart Association studies show that after a heart attack, patients with low social support are more likely to have symptoms of depression and low quality of life. A study in the United Kingdom revealed a similar scenario to that found in the Swedish and United States studies. They reviewed large prospective populations, which means they tracked them over a period of time. They adjusted for their social strata, risk factors, ethnicity, and age. Researchers found that those with loneliness and social isolation were more likely to experience their first heart attack and first stroke. Similarly, a Danish study revealed a 20% increased risk of developing cardiovascular disease with those who experienced loneliness. There was a 23% increased risk with those who were socially isolated for developing cardiovascular disease.

The Gut Microbiome

Our bodies are filled with trillions of bacteria. The collection of these organisms is known as the microbiome. While some bacteria are associated with disease, others work to strengthen our immune system and our heart, stabilize our weight, and support other health aspects. This reminds me of the movie

Venom. In the movie, there is an alien species that comes to earth looking for host bodies. The alien will be absorbed by the host human, but if there's no compatibility, the human will die. If the alien and the human are well matched, it gives the human superpowers. The aliens and humans work synergistically to fight crime. In a similar way, we have good species and bad species of microflora. The good bacteria work synergistically for our well-being, and the bad bacteria precipitate disease. We have more bacterial cells in our bodies than human cells. There are roughly 40 trillion bacterial cells in our bodies and only 30 trillion human cells. We are more living bacteria than we are living humans.

Within the human gut microbiome, a complex ecosystem teeming with around 1,000 different bacterial species, each microbe has a unique role to play. Recent scientific findings have unveiled a compelling connection between psychosocial stress, particularly the stress associated with loneliness, and its potential influence on cardiovascular disease through microbiome alterations. This stress-induced cascade not only activates our immune response but also diminishes microbiome diversity, creating a troubling cycle of stress begetting more stress. In essence, diversity within our gut bacteria is akin to strength, a principle applicable to nations, our global community, and, significantly, our own bodies. Greater bacterial diversity correlates with enhanced resilience and longevity. When we experience chronic stress, our body's stress response mechanisms can provoke disturbances in the gut microbiome, potentially leading to digestive problems and compromised immune function. Conversely, the power of intimacy within relationships can wield a profound impact on maintaining a well-balanced gut microbiome. Strong social connections and close emotional bonds have the capacity to alleviate stress and foster emotional well-being. Feeling emotionally supported and connected to others can foster a positive influence on our gut health. Extensive research suggests that positive social interactions and emotional intimacy contribute to sustaining a diverse and harmonious gut microbiome, thus promoting overall health and well-being. Therefore, while stress may disrupt our gut microbiome, nurturing intimate relationships serves as a potent tool for preserving its equilibrium and bolstering our physical and mental health.

Scientists are looking more extensively into a specific area of DNA called the epigenome. I simplistically describe the epigenome as a light switch because it turns DNA signals on and off. We oftentimes think that our DNA is our destiny, but scientists no longer believe that is the case. Lifestyle influences our DNA. A 1990s scientist from Duke University named Randy Jirtel, Ph.D, discovered that DNA is not the sole driver of our health. DNA is malleable. Jirtle practically stumbled into this revelation when playing around with agouti mice's diet. Agouti mice are naturally obese. They are yellow and prone to contract diabetes and cancer. When bred, they always gave birth to obese yellow mice. He started feeding the mothers vegetables and vegetable-enriched food pellets. The agouti mice gave birth to small brown mice, not obese yellow mice. This was a revolutionary discovery. This birthed the idea that our DNA is not our destiny. When we look at the epigenome, the areas on the DNA that determine how the DNA expresses, we find that they are influenced by our actions, our food, our stress levels, our sleep, and our activities. In short, what we do makes changes that affect the regulation of gene expression. In exploring various biological pathways, it becomes evident that addressing stress and loneliness can induce epigenetic changes with far-reaching consequences for our well-being. Notably, these epigenetic modifications have the potential to be inherited by future generations. Emerging evidence suggests that the stress and trauma experienced by one generation can be transmitted to subsequent ones, highlighting the profound impact of our experiences on the genetic legacy we pass on.

Loneliness and Dementia

I often see elderly patients. I noticed that cognitive decline followed social upheaval, such as when they had to live alone or their families moved away. I observed the relationship between social isolation and loneliness in the development of memory impairment, dementia, and other related types of dementia. My findings were not unique to me. Researchers, after keeping a close eye on a group of people for more than 10 years, found that feeling lonely was linked to a higher risk of developing dementia, a type of brain disease that affects memory and thinking skills. This risk was three times higher in people who were not usually at high risk for dementia because of their age and genes, which includes most people in the United States. Feeling lonely was also tied to poorer brain health markers, which could make a person more vulnerable to Alzheimer's disease and related types of dementias. The CDC reports that social isolation and loneliness are associated with a 50% increased risk of dementia. In 2016, scientists reported a novel association of loneliness with cortical amyloid burden in cognitively normal older adults, suggesting that loneliness is a neuropsychiatric symptom relevant to preclinical Alzheimer's disease. The higher our loneliness, the poorer our mental health and higher our risk for dementia. The intimacy of relationships matters.

Loneliness and Social Isolation in Viral Infections

The connection between loneliness, isolation, and vulnerability to viral illnesses existed well before the 2020 pandemic. In a particular study, researchers aimed to determine whether loneliness or social isolation posed a greater risk for cold symptoms independently. To do this, they enrolled 200 healthy individuals and administered surveys to assess loneliness levels and social connectivity. Following this, participants were exposed to rhinovirus 39, a common cold virus, via nasal drops and were quarantined for five days while reporting any cold symptoms experienced. Additionally, researchers monitored participants for chills and fevers based on their actual body temperatures. The findings suggested that feelings of loneliness were more strongly associated with self-reported illness symptoms than objectively measured social isolation. This implies that individuals who perceive themselves as lonely, regardless of their social circumstances, may be at a higher risk of developing cold symptoms.

Another study looked at loneliness and the response to viral vaccinations. Vaccinations are a hot topic. This compels us to ask this pertinent question: Is the vaccination equally as beneficial to individuals with perceived loneliness? Researchers checked the body's response to the influenza vaccination in 83 first semester, healthy university freshmen. They found that elevated levels of loneliness throughout the semester, along with small social networks (meaning they were socially isolated) were associated with a poor body immune response to the vaccination. Essentially, the more loneliness, the less effective the vaccination. Those who had both loneliness and social isolation were the least likely to have a favorable response to the vaccination.

Loneliness and Diabetes

It's not surprising that people who feel socially isolated and lonely are more likely to develop diabetes. This chapter highlighted how the desire for social interaction often mirrors food cravings. Additionally, high-stress situations can lead to increased cravings for fatty and sugary foods, which significantly raise the risk of diabetes when consumed in excess. Moreover, feelings of loneliness may lead to decreased exercise and disrupted sleep patterns, further increasing the risk of developing diabetes. When we consider all these factors together, it becomes clear how loneliness is closely linked to our behaviors and, ultimately, to diabetes.

A 20-year follow-up study with individuals who felt lonely

showed a two-fold higher risk of developing type 2 diabetes compared to those who did not feel lonely. We can also find a relationship between loneliness and social isolation with cancer. Together, they were associated with a higher total cancer incidence later in life. Loneliness and social isolation were associated with a higher risk of lung cancer as well. Being single was connected with poorer survival outcomes for cancer patients. The research confirms that social connectivity is crucial to our overall health.

The Power of Positive Relationships, Friendships, and Stress Hormones

We've seen how social isolation wreaks havoc on our health, now let's look at how healthy support systems benefit us. Studies confirm that individuals who have support systems are more likely to survive a heart attack and less likely to have recurrent heart attacks. So, there is a secret sauce in positive relationships. It's the same for married couples. People who have someone they can confide in are healthier. Strong relationships support our health. And so, the old saying that *a problem shared is a problem halved* is scientifically supported through clinical research. A California-based study found that the best way to beat stress is to share your feelings. Sharing thoughts and feelings with someone who has been in the same situation or shared a similar trauma proves to be the most effective way to relieve stress.

One study took a look at 52 female undergraduates. They paired participants and asked them to make a speech while being recorded by researchers. Take into consideration that public speaking, especially in front of others, triggers stress. Prior to each speech, part of the participants were encouraged to discuss how they felt about public speaking with researchers and their fellow participants. Other participants were told not to say anything, not to express their feelings. The cortisol levels of all the participants were measured before, during, and after each speech. Findings revealed that stress levels were significantly reduced when the participants were able to talk about how they felt about making the speeches. And the stress reduction was most noticeable when each participant shared a common fear. This brings us back to the effects of oxytocin, the love hormone and antithesis to the stress hormone which triggers fight or flight. Oxytocin drives us to come together to express shared experiences and to tend and befriend. How does this play a role in terms of disease outcome? There was a 2010 meta-analysis that looked at over 300,000 individuals taken from 148 studies that found that the likelihood of being alive is 50% higher for those with the strongest social relationships compared to people without such ties. So, as a predictor of survival, this is on par with the effect of quitting smoking. As an interventional cardiologist, I understand the health effects of smoking and how vital it is to stop smoking. So much so that it is a national quality metric to ensure that cardiologists counsel patients on smoking cessation. Stopping smoking can reduce a patient's risk of death by 50%. When we look at the relationship of the data on social ties and connections, doctors should also be asking patients about their social support, because studies tell us that the likelihood of survival is 50% greater with those who have significant social support. This same study found that people in happy marriages have lower blood pressure than people who weren't married. But people in strained marriages fare worse than single people. It's not just about getting together with someone, so don't take this as advice to marry anybody. Being in a bad relationship is toxic to both mind and body. You want to be involved with individuals that you can confide in, with whom you can share experiences, and who can empathize with you, as well as express care and concern for you. You need someone who speaks your love language.

One theory is that good relationships calm people down regarding the fight or flight response, the reaction that kicks in when we are scared or angry. Harvard Medical School psychiatrist and professor Dr. Waldinger says that the stress hormones released at such moments can be harmful. If you have a lousy day and go home and you have someone to talk with about it, you can feel your body decompress as you talk about what's gone wrong. You will experience even better results if your friend or partner is a good listener and offers encouragement.

The Power of Touch

I remember when my son was born. I would often put him to sleep, and my wife would read and lie with our daughter. In order to get him to calm down and sleep, I quickly learned that holding him close and kissing his cheek would relax him and cause him to rest. Scientists have discovered that our sense of touch begins to develop in the womb at around 14 weeks, and once we are born, being gently touched by a mother (or father) has numerous health benefits, including reducing heart rate and promoting the growth of brain cell connections. When someone hugs us, the stimulation of specific nerves in our skin sends signals to our brain's emotion processing networks, triggering a cascade of neurochemicals with proven health benefits. These include oxytocin, a hormone that promotes social bonding, slows heart rate, and reduces stress and anxiety, as well as endorphins in the brain's reward pathways, which create feelings of pleasure and well-being. Self-touching, such as placing a hand on the heart, activates memories of support and compassion.

In an experiment published in 2020, researchers wanted to see if physical touch could reduce feelings of loneliness, even in a culture where physical touch is not very common. The researchers did a study with 40 participants, and they found that when people were given physical contact, like a hug or a pat on the back, they reported feeling less lonely, especially if they were single. They also noticed that their heart rate went down, which is a sign of feeling better physically. These findings show that even though culture may not encourage a lot of physical touch, it can still help people feel less lonely.

In another physical touch study performed in 2021, researchers assessed the effects of self-soothing touch and receiving a hug on stress responses. They investigated in 159 healthy participants aged 18-35 years, who were exposed to a standardized psychosocial stressor. The study found that both self-soothing touch and receiving a hug had a significant effect on reducing cortisol levels, but not on heart rates or self-reported measures of stress. The study suggests that self-soothing touch and receiving hugs are simple yet potentially powerful means for individuals to cope with stress. Authors concluded when physical touch from others is limited (like what was experienced during the pandemic), self-soothing touch may be a useful alternative to reduce stress.

Other studies showed that men who have no contact with family and friends, compared to men who socialize with family and friends, frequently have increased risks of heart failure. Although the prior study tells us that women who were embraced had a reduction in cortisol levels, this study tells us that men can get value from contact with family and friends. These interactions lower their risk of heart failure.

A joint effort between researchers from Montreal University and Rush University Medical Center in Chicago conducted a comparative study of students and how they socially integrated into the campus community. Montreal University researchers recruited 60 international students who had just arrived in Canada. Each student had no friends, family, or romantic relationships in the area. They measured their heart rates and scheduled follow-up appointments two and five months later. Participants answered questions pertaining to their social lives and reported how many people they saw and talked to at least once a week. The study found that how well students integrated socially was associated with changes in heart rate variability. Heart rate variability (HRV) is the variation in the time interval between heartbeats. HRV is measured by the variation in the beat-to-beat interval. A shorter span of heart rate variability indicates the level of stress. When stress weighs you down, it weighs the heart down as well. An unstressed heart has a wide range of fluctuation. Participants who had minimal heart rate variability were more inclined to have increased stress levels. In another study, children who hung out with their best friends during a stressful situation had lower levels of cortisol over time as compared with children who were not able to hang out with their friends.

The Power of Companion Animals to Combat Loneliness

My daughter once asked my mother who her favorite child was, assuming it would be me, her youngest son, since my mom lives with me. However, my mom surprised her by answering "Precious" without hesitation. Precious is my mom's dog, which my sister bought for her after my dad passed away. Precious has been an important companion for my mom, seemingly sensing her moods and motivating her to exercise and socialize. Studies have shown that pet ownership can lead to greater well-being, self-esteem, and exercise and can also provide social support that complements human relationships. Pets can even help stave off negativity caused by social rejection. Overall, pets can provide important psychological and physical benefits for their owners.

The Power of Community

Friendships and social relationships are the core components of a community. So often we are isolated because we live and work inside our own silence. These are the periods of time in which we are socially isolated, physically isolated, and feel lonely. We have spoken many times already about the burden of disease that ensues from loneliness. We understand that it's important to establish a community, but many people don't know how to do this. There's no better example of interdependence within a community than that of the cooperation of trees. Yes, I said trees. Yes, those things that stand and don't move unless the wind blows them. Those things that seem inanimate, those objects that small animals climb and that produce fruit. Those things we call trees. They seem to live in isolation, but trees are survivalists. They survive crises and they help neighboring trees to do the same because they are rooted in community. Although they look like solitary individuals above ground, underground, we see a much different picture. Below ground, there is a vast community of roots and fungi. These trees are far from loners. Trees grow as a tight-knit group. They're intertwined. They're intermingled at their root level. They may seem like the tall silent type, but trees communicate. Only recently did scientists realize that trees talk with each other. I don't mean like in a Disney animated style where they talk aloud. No, they communicate through carbon, water, and nutrients. This is forest talk, and the conversation is transmitted through a network of fungi called the mycorrhizal network. It's an underground internet that's built by soil and fungi. Some jovially call this the wood wide web, the WWW. The WWW depends on trees that form vast social networks. The older trees are like older members of our community. Our elders convey their knowledge and experiences to the younger generation to ensure survival and betterment for the future. In the forest, the older trees do the same. They are referred to as mother trees, and they are the community cornerstones. They share extra nutrients with the younger ones when necessary. And if two trees are friends or they are the same type of tree, they help keep their branches from growing in each other's way. They can regulate their environment, air temperatures, and humidity, all of which are vital for their survival. Their roots are interconnected, and when one tree dies, the remaining trees often get sick. You might think that their social networks would collapse, but they don't. The miracle is that dying trees, even dead trees, continue to be part of the forest community. When the tree falls victim to natural disaster or disease, it can warn its neighbors through the WWW so they don't meet the same fate.

When trees are cut, they send signals, and the stumps that are still connected by their roots continue to share their resources to help the forest flourish. Scientists say that our forests, just like the rest of the world, are rooted in relationships.

Just like trees in a forest, when a family member passes away, the remaining family members, along with their friends, share resources. People bring food, send flowers, and provide comforting words to family members. There's power in interconnectivity, and although we are individuals, we are connected to our family, to our environment, and to our neighbors. These connections give us shared resources, provide power to members, and strengthen our community. This power helps us keep and maintain our health, minimize our stress levels, share our failures and successes, and subsequently achieve great things.

The Roseto community in eastern Pennsylvania gives us an example of a community where lifestyle parallels the activity and networking of our forests. Roseto was settled by immigrants from southern Italy in the late 1800s. For decades, people from Roseto maintained and protected their traditions and lifestyles from the old country. The town gained notoriety because the close-knit Italian American community exhibited half the national average rate of heart disease in the mid-20th century. Researchers call this the Roseto Effect. One example comes from the nearby town of Bangor, where there were 79 heart attacks from 1935 to 1944 compared to just 9 in Roseto. Though the two towns were only a mile apart, they continued to show the same dramatic disparity in congestive heart failure and overall death rates for decades. When the scientists looked at their Framingham Risk Score, looking at things like smoking, cholesterol, diabetes, weight, and exercise, they were unable to explain the difference. It wasn't as if their lifestyles were similar to those who lived in blue zones. One blue zone based in Loma Linda, CA, was made up of people who ate a plant-based diet, exercised, lived with purpose, and led spiritually well-rounded lives. No, Roseto residents smoked cigars, worked in metal casting factories, were exposed to airborne toxins, fried their meatballs, and ate foods like cheese and salami with abandon. But life in Roseto was different than life in surrounding areas. The grandparents lived with the grandchildren just like the mother trees in the forest. Many households had three or four generations living under the same roof. There were community-wide celebrations for life cycle events, and they were devoted churchgoers. Elders were revered and were an integral part of the community. No one was ever alone or lonely. Everyone had overwhelming support. There was no crime, no locked doors, no need for social welfare because the people took care of their own. But slowly, there was an integration of the standard American diet and the standard American lifestyle. People began to work long hours; they became more and more socially isolated. These changes produced a significant increase in the rate of heart attacks and deaths due to coronary artery disease. Roseto residents now suffer the same chronic diseases that most Americans suffer from.

The Roseto community as it operated in its early days and the cooperative spirit of our forest systems provide potent examples of life-enhancing relationships. While we may not be able to replicate them, we can do as much as possible to reach out to others, to form community, and to join with existing communities. There are always changes we can make in our lives, but as we can see from Roseto, eating better and exercising alone are not enough. Joining with others may be just the kickstart you need to live a healthier and happier life.

Becoming a part of a social community can be a fulfilling and enriching experience. To join such a community, it's important to take a few key steps. First and foremost, identify your interests and passions, as this will guide you toward a community that aligns with your values. Next, seek out local clubs, organizations, or online groups that share these interests. Attend meetings or events to meet like-minded individuals who share your enthusiasm. Actively engage and participate in group activities, discussions, and initiatives, as this will help you form connections and build relationships. Be open to new experiences and friendships, and don't hesitate to initiate conversations and reach out to others. Remember that community involvement is a two-way street, and your active participation will contribute to the group's overall cohesion and success.

For those who may not have access to a physical community and are unable to adopt a pet, I am excited to offer an opportunity to be a part of a growing online community, at www.DrBatiste.com that is focused on getting #SELFISH. The goal of this virtual community is to create a safe space that allows individuals from diverse backgrounds who are dedicated to fostering self-improvement, personal growth, and well-being to connect. In our online community, we encourage open discussions, share valuable resources, and provide support to help members embark on their journey to self-discovery and empowerment. By engaging with like-minded individuals online, you can still experience the sense of belonging and camaraderie that comes from being part of a community, even in the absence of physical presence. Together, we can embrace the #SELFISH philosophy and work toward becoming the best versions of ourselves.

CHAPTER 7

Sleep

I have always had a very interesting relationship with sleep. My first lesson about the importance of sleep came through observational learning during my childhood. As a child I remember being afraid of not only the dark but also being alone. I think I spent my first decade sleeping in my parents' room just so I could be near them. I remember my dad working at night as a probation officer, and during the day, he was doing everything from overseeing our family-owned pre school and teaching college courses to a variety of business ventures. It seemed as if he never slept. On the days when he wasn't working the night shift, I would often see him in his office or in the chair by his bed with the night lamp reading or working on new business strategies.

These early childhood experiences subconsciously shaped my impression of the importance of sleep. My dad was clearly a night owl, and despite my efforts to mimic his sleep pattern, I could never stay up late. Somehow, I would always wake up early. I later learned the reason why: chronotype.

A chronotype is like a personal clock that decides when we feel most active and awake. It's not something we can choose; it's determined by our genes, which are like our body's instructions. There are three main types: morning people, evening people, and in-between people.

Morning people like to wake up early in the morning, while evening people prefer to stay up late at night. Scientists have found that there are special genes that affect our chronotypes. Around a quarter to a third of people are evening types, another quarter to a third are morning types, and the rest are in-between. Our chronotype is related to our body's internal clock called the circadian rhythm. This rhythm lasts for 24 hours and controls when we sleep and wake up.

Even though everyone's circadian rhythm is similar, our chronotypes make our energy peaks happen at different times. For example, a morning person feels most awake in the early morning, while an evening person feels most alert in the evening. Because our chronotypes are different, we have different preferences for waking up and going to bed. A morning person might like to wake up around 5:30 a.m. and go to bed around 9:00 p.m., while an in-between person might wake up at 7:00 a.m. and go to sleep around 10:30 p.m.

I am a morning person, but I remember I tried to be someone I wasn't in medical school. In today's vernacular, I wasn't living my truth. Medical school is a unique experience because the sheer volume of information that one needs to learn is often compared to trying to drink water from a fire hydrant. I vividly remember my first year in medical school when an overwhelming sense of stress and apprehension washed over me while preparing for an exam. I realized I couldn't possibly "drink enough water," meaning I wasn't adequately prepared, and I was stressed (remember that stress = demands – resources). I knew I lacked a thorough understanding of the material, and time, an invaluable resource, was running out. So, I fell back on one of my earliest lessons from watching my father stay up late to get things done, and I knew what I had to do: Stay up all night and study.

The following day was a complete disaster. It felt as if I hadn't studied at all. My ability to recall information was impaired, my focus disappeared, and I struggled not only to comprehend the exam questions but also to provide coherent answers. Despite managing to pass the test, the lesson I learned had little to do with the actual content or subject matter. I discovered that beyond chronotype and being labeled as an early bird or a night owl, sleep plays an essential role in memory and performance. Getting adequate sleep, irrespective of your personal chronotype, is non-negotiable.

That medical school test became my personal experiment to evaluate the impact of sleep on learning. I later realized that learning is closely intertwined with a concept called neuroplasticity.

Neuroplasticity is a complex term that describes the brain's remarkable ability to change and grow when we learn new things. Just like how clay can be molded into different shapes, our brains can change and grow based on our experiences and what we learn. It's like a muscle that can get stronger with exercise.

When we learn new things or practice a skill, our brains create new connections between the cells called neurons. These connections help us remember information and perform tasks better. The more we practice or learn, the stronger these connections become.

Plasticity also means that our brains can recover from injuries or adapt to changes. For example, if someone hurts their arm and can't use it for a while, their brain might start using other parts of the body to help with tasks. Over time, the brain can even rewire itself to regain some of the lost abilities.

So, plasticity is like the brain's superpower that allows it to change, grow, and adapt based on our experiences and needs. It helps us learn new things, get better at skills, and recover from injuries. Our brains are amazing and flexible, just like clay that can be shaped into many different forms!

Neuroplasticity is not confined to specific stages of life but occurs throughout our lifespan. This means that learning is possible at any age, and the brain can continuously change and adapt in response to new experiences and information.

The brain, with its myriad of intricate tasks, is truly remarkable. What I hadn't realized in medical school is that during sleep, our brains are highly active, engaging in various processes that aid in learning, memory consolidation, and information retention. While we sleep, our brains undergo a process called synaptic plasticity, which is a fundamental mechanism of neuroplasticity. During this process, the connections between neurons, known as synapses, are strengthened or weakened based on our waking experiences and the information we encounter. Throughout sleep, the brain consolidates and integrates the acquired information from the day, reinforcing vital connections and eliminating unnecessary ones, essentially organizing and optimizing its neural networks. This process helps solidify memories and enhances learning. Therefore, my experiment on the impact of sleep deprivation on learning, despite passing the test, served as a demonstration that all-nighters do not aid in true learning.

That experience in medical school was only the beginning of my flirtation with an understanding of sleep. Over the years, I have taken an interest in the science of sleep, so much so that by the time I began to take care of Angie, I had incorporated sleep into my conversations with patients.

Once we are asleep, sleep plays a very important role in the regulation of our body function through hormone regulation. Recall how hormones are special chemicals in our bodies that help regulate various functions. When we sleep, our bodies produce and release different hormones that are important for our growth, development, and overall well-being. These hormones are like messengers telling different body parts what to do. One crucial hormone that gets released during sleep is growth hormone. It helps us grow taller and stronger and promotes the repair and regeneration of our cells and tissues. Another hormone affected by sleep is cortisol, the stress hormone. During sleep, cortisol levels decrease, which helps us feel more relaxed and less stressed. On the other hand, when we don't get enough sleep, cortisol levels can increase, making us feel more anxious and irritable. Sleep also influences the production of hormones that control our appetite and metabolism. Leptin and ghrelin are two hormones involved in regulating hunger and fullness. When we don't sleep enough, the balance of these hormones can be disrupted, leading to increased feelings of hunger and a higher risk of overeating. Sleep plays a role in the regulation of insulin, a hormone that helps control blood sugar levels. Lack of sleep can make it harder for our bodies to properly use insulin, which increases the risk of developing conditions like diabetes. In addition to playing a role in hormone regulation, sleep also impacts our immune system and our emotional health.

There are different stages or components to sleep. When we work out, we warm up by stretching or slowly jogging, we exercise, and then we cool down. The different phases of a workout are like the phases of sleep. First, we enter light sleep, similar to a warmup for physical exercise. This is the transition stage between wakefulness and sleep. As sleep progresses, we go into deeper periods of non-rapid eye movement, or NREM. You become less aware of your surroundings, your body temperature drops, your eye movements stop, and your breathing and heart rate become more regular. When you move into phase three, another level of NREM, your muscles completely relax, your blood pressure drops, breathing slows, and you progress into your deepest sleep known as the delta level. Finally, we enter phase four, REM, or rapid eye movement. This is the place where brain activity increases, the eyes move rapidly, the body is completely relaxed, you breathe faster, and you dream. It is harder to wake us during this phase because we are sound asleep. Sleep occurs in a series of recurring sleep stages that generally last from 90 to 110 minutes. Once we complete the first cycle, the subsequent cycles are not linearly progressive. Each sleep stage has a unique function and role in maintaining your brain's overall cognitive performance.

The REM stage is considered essential for the brain, enabling key functions such as growth hormone secretion and the release of other hormones important for metabolism. My wife and I used to tell my son that if he wanted to grow tall, he needed a good night's rest. Though we were joking, our jesting contained a bit of truth. Naturally, we encourage good nutrition because good health relies on a multitude of factors. Certainly, sleep and nutrition play an important role in a person's ability to regulate hormone secretion and to provide the proper nutrients to our bodies. During REM sleep, the autonomic nervous system activity, which is critical in regulating cardiovascular function, varies with sleep stages. It fluctuates with the parasympathetic system tone. The parasympathetic tone is the highest during that third stage of sleep, and sympathetic activation is highest during the REM sleep. If one never gets into that third stage, the parasympathetic tone never activates. The parasympathetic tone is the opposite of sympathetic tone. The parasympathetic tone allows the vessels to dilate, which can lower our blood pressure and reduce our heart rate. This allows our hearts to slow down and rest. Simply put, it calms us down. The sympathetic tone refers to the fight or flight neural activation. This activation prepares us for action. We need sleep to activate our parasympathetic tone.

The Causes and Issues with Sleep Disturbance

"How is your sleep?" I asked Angie during one of our weekly

check-ins. She hesitantly admitted that she hadn't been sleeping well. She described trouble both falling and staying asleep. Angie described her own turbulent relationship with sleep that began before the pandemic as she found herself attempting to balance life as a wife, mother, and business owner. Since the pandemic, Angie noted that her relationship with sleep seemed to fall apart like the other aspects of her life. She made the connection that the higher her stress, the poorer her sleep (sleep = resiliency/stress).

Angie's experience is, unfortunately, not unique. There are many reasons for sleep disturbances, but irrespective of the cause, the result is disruption of the body's natural cycle of sleep and wakefulness. Short-term, or acute, sleep disturbance can be caused by life stresses (job loss or death of a loved one), illness, or environmental factors (light, noise, extreme temperatures). Long-term sleep disturbance can be caused by depression, chronic stress, or pain or discomfort at night.

When we're awake, our brains produce a chemical called adenosine. It builds up in our brains throughout the day. But when we sleep, this chemical is cleared out. Adenosine helps us feel sleepy and promotes sleep in our brains. Normally, it takes about 8 hours of sleep to completely remove adenosine from our brains. However, when a person doesn't get enough sleep, they may never feel fully awake during the daytime. It's like their brain is always a little sleepy. Daytime sleepiness refers to feeling excessively tired or drowsy during the daytime when we are supposed to be awake and active.

Daytime sleepiness is related to a sleep disturbance or an inability to achieve adequate sleep. When we have inadequate sleep, our brain also reacts by making us less alert and causing something called microsleep. Microsleep is when we briefly fall asleep for just a few seconds, even though our eyes may still be open. During these short episodes, our brains don't process information, and we may experience lapses in attention.

Numerous studies have highlighted the impact of sleep deprivation on the medical community. These studies indicate that health professionals who experience different levels of sleep-related impairment, ranging from moderate to very high, are more likely to self-report medical errors. Specifically, when compared to individuals with low sleep-related impairment, those with moderate, high, and very high sleep-related impairment had significantly higher odds of making medical errors, with the odds being 53%, 96%, and 97% greater, respectively. These findings emphasize the crucial importance of addressing sleep-related issues in healthcare to reduce the risk of medical errors and ensure safer patient care.

Research, which explored the connection between fatigue induced by sleep deprivation and the clinical performance of medical residents, played a central role in driving the graduate medical education body to implement more stringent regulations regarding the maximum consecutive hours physicians in training could work. In 2005, the medical board introduced new guidelines that limited residents to 80 working hours per week, prohibited them from working more than 24 consecutive hours during a single duty shift, and mandated that they could not be on call more frequently than every third night, with at least one day off each week. However, this significant decision was made after my own training. Reflecting on my time as a resident, it often felt as though I was expected to achieve the impossible, all while contending with severe sleep deprivation. During clinical rounds, I struggled to remain alert and devised various strategies to maintain organization. I meticulously maintained alphabetically arranged notebooks containing patient information, frequently creating charts and to-do lists to refine my processes. This meticulous record-keeping was essential because I recognized that sleep deprivation increased the likelihood of errors. This approach enabled me to deliver effective care for my patients, ensuring that even during sleepless nights, I wouldn't overlook critical details.

Numerous studies have drawn parallels between the cognitive and physiological impairments caused by fatigue and those induced by alcohol intoxication. In essence, not getting enough sleep can be likened to being under the influence of alcohol. One study, for instance, compared the performance of individuals who had been awake for 17 hours to those with a specific blood alcohol concentration. The findings suggested that staying awake for 17 hours is akin to having a blood alcohol concentration of approximately 0.05% and being awake for a full 24 hours is similar to having a blood alcohol concentration of around 0.1%. In the United States, the legal limit for blood alcohol concentration when operating a vehicle is defined as 0.08% or higher. However, impaired driving can be observed at blood alcohol concentrations as low as 0.05%. Some countries have even set their cutoff at 0.05% or lower for driving purposes. A survey published in the journal *Anesthesia* in 2017 revealed that 57% of healthcare respondents had experienced accidents or near misses when commuting home after night shifts. When we fail to obtain adequate sleep, our judgment becomes compromised, particularly when it comes to driving, putting ourselves and others at grave risk. Reflecting on my years of medical training, I consider myself fortunate to have avoided any major car accidents. There were instances when, utterly drained mentally, I'd leave the hospital and drive home, encountering brief episodes of microsleep where I'd inadvertently doze off for a few seconds at the same stoplight.

Increased Sleep Disturbance During COVID

Angie grappled with worsened sleep issues during the COVID-19 pandemic, but she found solace in knowing that her struggle was not unique. The pandemic's global impact was far-reaching, prompting an extensive examination of sleep disruptions that spanned from November 1, 2019, to July 15, 2021, coinciding with the peak of the crisis. This thorough analysis encompassed 250 studies involving half a million participants from fifty different countries. The results revealed a worldwide prevalence of sleep disturbances at around 40.49%, with notably higher rates occurring during lockdown periods, when it surged to nearly 43%, as opposed to 38% during non-lockdown periods. It was disclosed that roughly four out of every ten individuals encountered sleep-related challenges during the pandemic, with the most severe effects observed in those afflicted by COVID, as well as in children and adolescents.

Additionally, scientists found a strong link between feeling more stressed, having higher anxiety, and experiencing changes in sleep patterns. They learned that self-esteem could help lessen how stress and anxiety affect sleep quality. Plus, how well you sleep can affect how stressed or anxious you feel. This complicated connection between stress and anxiety keeps going in a circle, where feeling more stressed and anxious leads to worse sleep, and bad sleep makes stress and mental health issues worse, making the cycle stronger.

I took the opportunity to explain to Angie that in addition to the sleep challenges she faced due to stress, her feelings of loneliness likely exacerbated her sleep issues. I cited a study that explored the consequences of loneliness and isolation, revealing that individuals experiencing loneliness, whether living alone or with others, were more prone to reporting sleep disturbances and related problems compared to those who did not experience loneliness.

The Impact of Stress on Sleep

Anything that activates the fight or flight system is a stressor. Adrenaline prepares us for danger. This is useful when we're running from a dog because we need that adrenaline to get going, but when it's happening regularly, and no dog is coming at us, it's harmful to our bodies. We live in a time when we can feel as if we are in the middle of a war zone just by watching a movie. Toxic relationships leave us waiting for the next shoe to drop, and we are triggered by numerous negative interactions.

As I have mentioned before, when we are repeatedly triggered, we set off a cascade of hormones that creates a stress response. It is almost impossible to sleep when we are stressed. We need to calm down so we can rest. Being stressed when we are trying to sleep is like trying to sleep when people in our homes are yelling because we can't settle down due to the noise. We need to turn off our thoughts so we can drift off, but with Angie, that was not the case. Her mind ran rampant about what happened, what could have been, what she could have done to prevent her circumstances, and how desolate her life was currently. She could not turn her mind off. She couldn't sleep. She was drained and stressed due to the lack of sleep, and she was stuck in a brutal cycle.

Researchers have extensively studied the connection between stress and sleep problems. They've found that when sleep is disturbed, it's often linked to various sources of psychological stress, such as academic pressure, difficult life events, work issues, financial problems, and discrimination. Other studies focus on stress that feels out of control and unpredictable. This kind of stress is what we talk about when we say stress equals demands minus resources. Sometimes we face demands that we just can't handle, like not having enough time or dealing with a natural disaster like a hurricane. When we're in these situations, it feels like we're stuck without the resources we need to cope, which causes a lot of stress. And when we feel like things are out of control, it's hard to sleep well.

High levels of stress can make it take longer to fall asleep and disrupt the quality of our sleep. This triggers our body's stress response system, leading to an increase in stress hormones like cortisol, which can make it even harder to sleep. When we're stressed, we might find ourselves lying awake at night, unable to relax. People who are stressed often complain about not getting enough sleep. It's clear that stress affects how well we sleep, but it works the other way around, too – when we don't sleep well, it can make us feel even more stressed.

One study was conducted to find out how many teenagers don't get enough sleep and if it affects their emotions and behavior. They also looked at how things like activities before bed and stress can affect how much sleep teenagers get. They asked a big group of teenagers in Sweden to fill out questionnaires during school. They found that 12% of younger teenagers (12-13 years old) and 18% of older teenagers (14-16 years old) didn't get enough sleep according to the new sleep guidelines. Those teenagers who didn't get enough sleep also had more problems with their behavior and emotions, like being depressed, anxious, or angry.

The study also found that teenagers who felt stressed at home or stressed about their school performance were more likely to not get enough sleep. And teenagers who did things like using their phones or computers in bed got less sleep, too. The researchers think that it's important to help teenagers have better sleep by addressing things like using technology before bed, stress, and worries. They want to find ways to help teenagers create good sleep habits and feel better emotionally.

As I discussed in the intimacy chapter, healthy interpersonal relationships offer safety, security, and connection. These feelings assist one's ability to fall and stay asleep. When we are safe, there is no need for hypervigilance because we can completely relax. Multiple studies document that couples in good relationships have fewer symptoms of insomnia. So obviously, the better your relationships, the better your sleep. The relationship between couples' sleep and the quality of their interactions appears to be linked; the more sleep the partners get, the better their interactions and the better their interactions, the better the quality of their sleep. Research tells us that when we nurture our relationships, we create a safe and stable climate for rest and sleep.

The Relationship Between Poor Sleep and Stress Hormones

In a well-rested state, cortisol, a hormone in the body, naturally decreases throughout the day. However, when you experience partial or total sleep deprivation, commonly known as sleep debt, your daytime cortisol levels can significantly increase, spiking by 37-45%. This happens because sleep, especially deep sleep, plays a crucial role in suppressing cortisol production. Therefore, inadequate sleep becomes a major contributor to heightened cortisol secretion. As an interventional cardiologist, I sometimes face sleep deprivation while attending to emergency cases. While my training has equipped me to remain functional, I've noticed that as I've grown older, recovery has become more challenging. A particularly alarming incident occurred after a night on call with less than 5 hours of fragmented sleep when I experienced chest discomfort and discovered my blood pressure was higher than usual. After a battery of tests, which thankfully yielded normal results, I realized the connection between these symptoms and my sleep patterns. When the body undergoes stress, it releases stress hormones. Therefore, it's confirmed that sleep deprivation leads to elevated stress hormone levels. A study from 1997 found that even missing a few hours of sleep for one night can raise cortisol levels the following evening. A 2021 study reaffirmed these findings, emphasizing that sleeping for 5 1/2 hours or less increases cortisol production in the afternoon and evening. These stress hormones immediately trigger a rapid increase in heart rate and blood pressure, potentially leading to symptoms like chest pain, sweating, and difficulty breathing.

Lack of sleep initiates a cycle in which sleep loss and excess cortisol mutually reinforce each other. Just one night of inadequate sleep can elevate your cortisol levels the following evening while also delaying cortisol production. The consequence of this cycle is elevated cortisol levels in your body, which persist even later in the day, further delaying your desired bedtime and reducing your total sleep duration. Consequently, your sleep debt continues to accumulate.

Furthermore, poor sleep acts as a stressor to the body, leading to the release of stress hormones and markers of inflammation. In a review of 72 studies, researchers established a link between sleep disturbances, including insomnia symptoms, and increased levels of inflammatory markers such as interleukin (IL)-6 and C-reactive protein (CRP). These markers are predictive of future heart-related events like heart attacks. In another study, scientists aimed to understand the relationships between sleep, pain, and inflammation in our bodies. They conducted a study with volunteers, with some sleeping only 4 hours a night for 10 days, while others slept for 8 hours a night. They measured certain substances in their blood and urine related to inflammation and assessed the volunteers' mood and pain levels throughout the study.

The results showed that volunteers who had less sleep had higher levels of IL-6 and CRP. Additionally, those with higher levels of IL-6 reported more pain when sleep-deprived. This indicates that insufficient sleep can exacerbate pain due to increased inflammation in our bodies. This is vital to understand because in certain medical conditions, individuals struggle with sleep, which can worsen their pain and inflammation.

There are other stress hormone responses triggered by poor sleep. During times of stress or sleep deprivation, our ghrelin levels can rise. Ghrelin is a hormone that signals when our body needs food, potentially providing extra energy to deal with stressful situations. It's like a signal telling our body, "We need to be ready to fight or flee!" Researchers have found that ghrelin levels increase when people experience physical stress, mental stress, or both together. This may explain why we tend to have increased cravings and experience the "munchies" when we are sleep deprived.

The Relationship Between the Amygdala and Sleep

In the realm of sleep, understanding how our brains function during rest is crucial. One key player in this story is the amygdala, a small but powerful part of the brain responsible for connecting memories with emotions, particularly those linked to fear. Think of it as the trigger for our fear response. Remember, it's why I become extremely scared of rats and mice. The amygdala, however, doesn't work alone; it's part of a larger system known as the limbic system, which assists us in managing intense emotions and storing memories.

Now, let's dive into the intriguing connection between sleep and our emotions. When we struggle to get enough sleep or experience sleep disturbances, it disrupts the communication between the amygdala and another important region called the ventral anterior cingulate cortex (VACC). This VACC acts like a control center for our emotions, helping us understand our feelings, empathize with others, and make decisions. Imagine it as a superhero inside our heads, aiding us in managing our emotions.

But here's the twist: When we're sleep-deprived, our brains struggle to regulate our emotions. The amygdala becomes hypersensitive to negative stimuli, causing us to feel more emotional and unstable. Typically, our thoughts are processed through the prefrontal cortex, another brain region that acts as a filter for our fears and helps us think rationally. It's how we navigate everyday challenges and make wise choices. This ability to reason and make good choices, however, diminishes when we're sleep deprived.

In essence, ensuring we get enough sleep is vital for our brains to function optimally. It enables our brains to act as the superhero inside our heads, maintaining emotional control and guiding us toward wise decisions in our daily lives. Just like how we need rest after a tiring day, our brains need rest to perform at their best!

Dr. Matthew Walker and colleagues from the University of California at Berkeley and Harvard Medical School examined how sleep loss affects the activation of the brain's amygdala. These researchers published a study in the 2007 issue of *Current Biology*. The study included 26 healthy individuals who were divided into two groups. One group had a normal night's sleep, and the other group was kept awake for 36 hours. Then each participant was given a functional magnetic resonance imaging (fMRI) scan as they viewed 100 different images. The initial images were emotionally neutral, but the images became increasingly unpleasant and disturbing. Participants viewed images such as dirty toilet bowls, burn victims, dying patients, or mutilated bodies. Both groups responded with greater amygdala activity, but the intensity and the volume of activation was 60% higher in the sleep-deprived group. This study demonstrates that we're more inclined to overreact when our sleep is disturbed or when we are sleep deprived and that not getting enough sleep is dangerous. When sleep deprived, we disrupt the brain's emotional safeguards. Getting a good night's sleep restores our emotional brain circuits and prepares us for the next day's challenges.

Another study looked at the relationship between anxiety and the amygdala's activity. Eighteen young adults watched emotionally stirring video clips after a full night's sleep and again after a sleepless night. Anxiety levels were measured following each session using a questionnaire and an MRI. After a night of no sleep, the participants showed a shutdown of the prefrontal cortex. You may remember that the prefrontal cortex is the part of the brain that processes information and keeps anxiety in check. The study also found that the brain's deeper emotional centers, like the amygdala, were overactive. Researchers concluded that sleep loss can casually and directionally instigate a high level of anxiety in those who are otherwise non clinically anxious when rested.

The Relationship Between Poor Sleep and Judgment

Researchers reveal that insufficient sleep or sleep disturbances contribute to aberrant behavior. Chronically sleep-restricted people exhibit increased bouts of risk-taking behavior. Lack of sleep or sleep disturbances may impair their reasoning faculties and cause jumping to conclusions without considering all the facts. In a study from 2001, scientists at the Walter Reed Army Institute of Research looked at how sleep deprivation affects decision-making. They had 26 healthy adults participate in the study. First, the participants were tested to see how well they made decisions about moral dilemmas when they were well rested. Then, they were tested again after going 53 hours without sleep.

The researchers found that when the participants were sleep-deprived, they took longer to make decisions. It was harder for them to figure out the best choice. This is similar to how I felt when I had to take a test after staying up all night studying. I was slower to respond, even if I knew the answers well.

Based on these findings, the researchers concluded that not getting enough sleep for a long time can make it difficult for our judgment and decision-making abilities to work correctly. These abilities rely on both thinking and feeling, and sleep deprivation can affect how well they work together.

Other researchers added to the narrative concerning sleep. Their data provided further support of the hypothesis that sleep loss is particularly disruptive to the brain's prefrontal cortex. The prefrontal cortex integrates affect and cognition, judgment, and decision making. Another 2010 study reported in the journal *Sleep* explored the impact of long-term partial sleep deprivation on the activation of moral justice and decisions. Researchers wanted to assess how not getting enough sleep for a long time affects people's moral judgments. Seventy-one naval and army officer cadets participated in the study. First, they were asked to judge 5 different scenarios when they were well-rested. Then, they were asked to do the same thing after not getting enough sleep for a while.

The results showed that when the officers were sleep-deprived, their ability to make mature and principled moral judgments was affected. They became more focused on following rules, but their ability to think about what's fair and just decreased. However, it didn't affect everyone the same way. Those who were already good at making mature moral judgments when rested lost that ability when sleep deprived, while those who weren't as good at it were not affected.

Scientists concluded that not getting enough sleep for a long time can affect how people make moral judgments. It can make them more focused on following rules and less able to think about what's fair and just.

More on Lack of Sleep and Hunger:

"Sleepy and Snacky: How Poor Sleep Makes Us Crave Junk Food!"

Angie and I had a conversation about how her sleep troubles seemed to be linked to weight gain. She noticed that the longer she stayed awake, the more she craved snacks. A *Scientific American* article quoted a study reporting that after two consecutive nights of four hours or less of sleep, the test subjects had a 28% higher level of ghrelin, the hunger hormone, and 18% lower leptin levels, the satiety hormone, compared with subjects who had 10 hours of sleep each night. The study stated that those who were sleep deprived self-reported that their hunger rating increased by 24% and their appetite rating increased by 23%.

I've noticed that the longer I'm up, the more I get the munchies. When I was in medical school, we had free access to the cafeteria, and if the cafeteria was closed, the nurse's station was always loaded with food. After staying up at all hours, we were tempted by a feast of ultra-processed foods. These foods became our comfort food. As you may remember, comfort food triggers our hunger. So here we were, sleep-deprived and eating junk foods. The lack of sleep increased our ghrelin levels while decreasing our leptin levels. Since food was everywhere, there was always an opportunity to eat. My colleagues and I were not the only ones to experience this increased desire for the standard American diet. A study conducted in Sweden in 2012 looked at how sleep affects our cravings for unhealthy food. The researchers found that when we don't get enough sleep, we tend to want more high-calorie junk food. They studied people who were not allowed to sleep as much as others and found that they reported feeling hungrier, and their brains showed stronger reactions to pictures of food. The study also showed that the longer we go without enough sleep, the stronger our desire for unhealthy food becomes. This can make us want to eat foods that add to our stress instead of our resiliency.

Research has shown that when people don't get enough sleep, they tend to eat more fatty foods like fried dishes and animal products. In addition, the hormone peptide YY, which tells our bodies when we're full after eating, decreases in people who have only had five hours of sleep for two consecutive nights. This suggests that when people are sleepy, they're not only more likely to eat comfort foods but also to eat more of them if given the chance.

Studies consistently show that high-stress levels are linked to eating more highly processed foods. We know that not getting enough sleep leads to stress, and stress makes us want to eat more and affects our hormones. These processed foods can also raise our perceived stress levels, which may increase the amount of cortisol in our bodies. When we eat these foods later in the day, when our bodies should be winding down, the increased cortisol levels can indirectly cause our bodies to store more fat and use muscle for energy. People who don't get enough sleep tend to lose more muscle and gain more fat compared to those who are well-rested.

In a study where participants followed a diet with 10% fewer calories for two weeks, those who slept for 5 1/2 hours each night lost 0.6 kilograms of fat and 2.4 kilograms of other tissues. On the other hand, those who got 8 1/2 hours of sleep each night lost 1.4 kilograms of fat and 1.5 kilograms of other tissues. This shows that there is a relationship between sleep and weight gain, as lack of sleep gives us more time to eat. Additionally, not getting enough sleep affects our prefrontal cortex, the part of our brain responsible for reasoning and willpower, making it harder to stick to our health goals. Lack of sleep also reduces our energy levels and changes our basal metabolic rate, which is the number of calories our bodies burn while at rest. Therefore, it may better to prioritize sleep over late-night exercise to reap the benefits.

The Relationship Between Poor Sleep and Cardiac Disease

It wasn't until 2015 that I truly grasped how sleep deprivation could affect heart health. In January of that year, CNN reported two tragic incidents at an internet café where gamers (people who play video games online) paid to play continuously for 72 and 120 hours. Shockingly, both individuals were found dead due to cardiac arrest caused by severe sleep deprivation. It was at this point that I began to delve deeply into the connection between poor sleep and its impact on heart health.

Scientific research has convincingly shown that both the duration and quality of sleep can have a significant influence on our health, potentially leading to early death and various adverse outcomes. One important study, the Sleep Heart Study, aimed to understand how insufficient sleep, including conditions like poor sleep quality, along with objectively measured short sleep duration, relate to cardiovascular disease and mortality. The findings revealed a 29% higher risk of cardiovascular disease in individuals with poor sleep coupled with inadequate sleep duration compared to those with regular sleep patterns. Moreover, poor sleep combined with objectively measured short sleep was associated with an elevated risk of cardiovascular events.

A study reported in the 2019 *Journal of American College of Cardiology* compared people who slept between 6 and 9 hours each night. It found that short sleepers had a 20% higher risk of heart attacks, while long sleepers had a 34% higher risk. The ideal amount of sleep, much like Goldilocks, is not too little or too much but around 7 to 9 hours, which is most beneficial for overall health.

Research into the timing of sleep onset has shown that individuals who go to bed at midnight or later face a 25% higher risk of cardiovascular disease, with a 12% greater risk for those who go to sleep between 11 p.m. and midnight. The quality of sleep varies throughout the night, with deeper non-rapid eye movement (non-REM) sleep occurring earlier and more rapid eye movement (REM) sleep as morning approaches. Both types of sleep are vital, but non-REM sleep is especially restorative, reducing cardiac stress. The transition from non-REM to REM sleep follows a specific schedule, meaning that going to bed very late, such as at 3 a.m., leads to less deep, restorative sleep. A comprehensive study conducted in the United Kingdom, spanning from 2006 to 2010 and involving 88,000 participants predominantly around 61 years old, examined sleep patterns and their relation to cardiovascular health over 5.7 years. The findings reaffirmed that individuals who slept after midnight had the highest rates of cardiovascular disease, while those who went to bed between 10 and 11 p.m. experienced the lowest rates of such issues.

Insomnia poses a risk to all aspects of heart health. Studies have shown that individuals with insomnia face an increased risk of heart failure, like Broken Heart Syndrome, where the heart doesn't squeeze as well. For example, a 2013 study found that heart failure risk was over threefold higher in insomniacs. Additionally, a 2021 study published in *The Journal of American*

College of Cardiology investigated the link between healthy sleep patterns and heart rhythm problems. It found that maintaining a good sleep pattern was associated with a 29% lower risk of atrial fibrillation/flutter (an irregular heartbeat) and a 35% lower risk of bradyarrhythmia (a slow heartbeat) compared to those with poor sleep habits.

In summary, sleep plays a critical role in heart health, and both the duration and timing of sleep can impact our cardiovascular well-being. Getting the right amount of quality sleep is like providing our hearts with a protective shield, reducing the risk of heart disease and related issues.

How a Lack of Sleep or Poor Sleep Leads to Cardiovascular Disease

Most people know that the autonomic nervous system is the way the body functions without our conscious control, but few know of the intricate workings within. When we dig deeper, we find what we call a parasympathetic tone. Parasympathetic tone is a network of nerves that relaxes the body after periods of stress or danger. It helps run life-sustaining processes like digestion during times when we feel safe and relaxed. When this parasympathetic activity decreases, sympathetic activity increases. The sympathetic nervous system is best known for its role in responding to dangerous or stressful situations. This increased activity is a risk factor for cardiovascular disease. To summarize, short sleep duration increases cardiovascular disease risks through autonomic dysfunction, meaning suppressing parasympathetic tone, and by increasing sympathetic activity. When this happens, the result is an increase in the variability of the heart beating and secretion of the hormone called norepinephrine.

One study looked at physicians who were on call and sleep deprived for 26 hours. Let's recall the meaning of the term heart rate variability (HRV). HRV refers to your **heartbeat's ability to shift beat to beat**. Imagine your heartbeats as musical notes in a song. Heart rate variability (HRV) is like the rhythm and tempo of that song. When your heart beats in a "staccato" pattern, it's like playing short, quick notes on a piano, one after the other, with little variation in the time between each note. This represents low HRV and can indicate heightened sympathetic tone. On the other hand, when your heart beats in a "legato" pattern, it's like playing long, flowing notes with some variations in the timing between them, creating a smoother and more harmonious melody. This indicates higher HRV, which is generally a sign of a lower sympathetic tone. So, HRV measures the variation in time between heartbeats, and a more "legato" pattern is a good sign for your overall well-being. Back to the study. Researchers focused on doctors who experienced 26 hours of being on call and sleep-deprived, examining their heart rate variability before and after this period of acute sleep deprivation. They found that even after just one night without sleep, their heart rate variability decreased, providing a real-life example of the impact of sleep deprivation on the body.

Another relationship between poor sleep and the occurrence of cardiovascular events finds its way through the highway of the body, the endothelium. This cellular layer that lines our vessels was identified as a port of entry for the COVID-19 virus. It is the same area where studies have shown is predictive of diabetes, high blood pressure, and many cardiovascular and chronic disease states. It's not surprising that literature reveals that sleep deprivation has an impact on endothelial function. Researchers examined cardiologists who were on call for 24 hours, and results showed an increase in blood pressure in 13 out of 15 physicians, which indicated poor endothelial function. It suggests that the difference in endothelial function is related to the stress from poor sleep. It is traditionally accepted that mental stress is linked to the sympathetic nervous system endothelial function. These physicians have double stress—stress from the lack of sleep as well as stress from making multitudes of complex medical decisions.

I regret to say that healthcare providers are not immune to the effects of insomnia; unfortunately, insomnia seems to affect even these healthcare superheroes. An observational study conducted in 2012 involved 22 healthy female nurses who worked three consecutive night shifts. The results revealed a decrease in flow-mediated dilatation, which assesses the endothelium's function and the arteries' ability to dilate—a greater ability to dilate indicates a healthier endothelium. The study demonstrated that endothelial function decreased from the baseline measured after sleepless shifts.

Similarly, another study involved 30 healthy physicians who had been working night shifts for an average of three to five years. Researchers assessed endothelium function after a regular workday to establish a baseline and then reexamined it after a continuous 24-hour workday. The findings showed a significant decrease in endothelium reactivity following shift work compared to the baseline measurements. These studies are just a small sample of numerous research efforts that suggest a link between shift work, sleep deprivation due to work-related stress, and vascular function.

How to Improve Sleep

After discussing research and my personal experiences, Angie asked, "I understand the importance, but how can I increase my sleep?" Let's get back to the basics: smart tools. As mentioned earlier, smart tools involve setting goals that are Specific, Measurable, Achievable, Relevant, and Time-bound (SMART). These tools can enhance various aspects of your life, and now we'll apply them to improving your sleep patterns. When we revisit the Selfish approach, we find that each aspect is applicable to enhancing our sleep quality as well.

The "S" in Selfish stands for spiritual. Studies show that when we relax and clear our minds, especially in the evening while taking a few moments for meditation and prayer, we improve our sleep. Research demonstrates that even people with insomnia can improve their sleep quality when they practice mindfulness meditation. Mindfulness meditation can serve as an auxiliary treatment for people who have sleep complaints. Let's learn how to apply our SMART tools. First, be specific about whether you want to focus on prayer or meditation. Think about how you'll measure your progress. Maybe you can use a helpful app or program. Make sure your goal is achievable and believe in yourself. Ask yourself if you're willing to give this a try and if prayer and meditation are relevant to your goals. Lastly, set a realistic time frame, like a month or six weeks, and use the workbook and outline to keep track of your approach. This way, you can work toward better sleep through spiritual practices.

Now, let's talk about the "E" in Self*fish*, which stands for exercise. Research from six different studies has shown that regular exercise can help improve sleep quality, especially for people in middle to older age groups. But there's something even better: exercising outdoors. When you exercise outside, you get to connect with nature and breathe in fresh air, which can also reduce feelings of sadness. Exposing yourself to morning sunlight during outdoor activities might even help reset your body's internal clock. However, it's important not to exercise too close to bedtime or late in the evening because it can make it harder to fall asleep. The best time to exercise is in the morning.

Now, when you decide to start exercising, think about what activities you enjoy. Do you like walking, dancing, doing sit-ups, or practicing yoga? You can even mix different exercises if you like variety. It's also helpful to set specific goals and measure your activity. There are apps and workbooks that can help you track your progress and stay motivated. Make sure you have everything you need for your chosen exercise, whether it's walking shoes or a yoga mat. And don't let rainy days stop you— you can find indoor activities, too. Decide how many days a week and how long you want to exercise and remember that exercise is indeed connected to your goal of better sleep. So, take a deep breath and know that you're on the right track to improving your sleep through exercise.

Next in the Selfish equation we have "L" for love. I spoke earlier about love being an action, so what action will you take? Love can come in the form of forgiveness, gratitude, and volunteering. We know these activities create oxytocin and that oxytocin has a positive impact on our mood. Studies show that gratitude improves sleep quality. To take advantage of that effect, write down three things that you're thankful for an hour before going to sleep. Studies show this action not only improves your outlook, it also improves your sleep quality. My wife gives love to herself when she takes a bath. She loves baths, but baths are not just an emotional booster; baths relax you and lower your core temperature when you emerge from the bathtub. Of course, use your smart tools to determine the actions you will take, when you will take them, how you will measure them, your time frames, and the relevancy.

The next letter in our Selfish plan is "F," which stands for food. It's essential to know that what you eat can affect your sleep, especially as we get older. Research tells us that having a meal or snacks close to bedtime can harm the quality of our sleep. So, try not to eat dinner or snacks too late in the evening. Also, it's a good idea to avoid caffeine in the evening because caffeine is a stimulant that can keep you awake. One study found that drinking caffeinated beverages six hours before bedtime can significantly make your sleep worse. Alcohol, while it might initially make you feel sleepy, can actually disrupt your sleep once its sedative effects wear off. It can mess with your sleep cycles and decrease the important REM sleep, which helps restore our bodies. Lastly, try to limit your liquid intake close to bedtime to avoid waking up in the middle of the night to use the bathroom, which can disturb your sleep. Remember, using the SMART approach can help you set specific, measurable, achievable, relevant, and time-based goals to improve your sleep habits.

The next letter in Self*ish* is "I," and it stands for intimacy, which means having close and supportive relationships. Studies have found that having people in your life who support and care for you is connected to better sleep quality, while negative relationships can lead to worse sleep. I've personally noticed that when my wife is away, I don't sleep well, and recent research confirms the importance of positive relationships for good sleep. A recent study in *Frontiers* discovered that married people tend to have more and better REM sleep compared to those who have never been married. So, it's clear that supportive relationships are linked to good sleep. However, it's not always easy to have supportive people around, which is why having a community, whether online or in person, is crucial. You need friends to talk to, socialize with, and connect with; people who share your goals and interests. As you look for opportunities to build relationships, be specific in your efforts. You could volunteer, be more open and friendly, or strengthen your existing friendships. Remember to make this step specific, measurable, achievable, relevant, and time-based to help you achieve better sleep and a happier life.

The second "S" in our Self*ish* plan is all about sleep, and it's crucial to give sleep a chance. Our bodies have their own routines, and they aim for a balanced state called homeostasis. To get the most out of our sleep, it's helpful to stick to a consistent sleep schedule: going to bed and waking up at the same time each day. You can make small, gradual changes to improve your sleep duration. For example, try going to bed 15 minutes earlier every night for three months, then increase that by a bit every three months over a year. Aim for around 7 to 9 hours of sleep each night. It's a good idea to limit daytime naps because they can affect the quality of your nighttime sleep. Also, if you have medical issues like obstructive sleep apnea or snoring, make sure to address them, as they can harm your health and longevity. Remember to set clear, achievable goals for better sleep—specific, measurable, doable, relevant, and with a timeframe in mind.

The last letter in Self*ish* is "H." The "H" stands for humor. Laughter is extremely important. Though we haven't touched on laughter yet, it's coming up in the next chapter. Meta analysis studies show that laughter and humor are effective in alleviating depression and anxiety and improving sleep quality in adults. You want to experience the joy of life. Research demonstrates that even a light chuckle is helpful. You can even *fake it 'til you make it*. Yes, even mild amusement and faking it have a positive effect on your outlook, body, and vasculature. Once more, take the smart approach to adding humor, joy, happiness, and laughter into your life.

CHAPTER 8

Humor

My clinic visits with my patients often end with a simple question: "When was the last time you laughed?" I can't recall when or why I started asking my patients this question. I wasn't prompted by a landmark medical study or by the movie Patch Adams, which I never saw. It was my intuition. After years of listening to patients and watching their body language, something even more profound than rapport surfaced. It got easier to hear what they said, the metacommunication that peeped through their words. My patients were joyless and stress filled. As I mentioned before, stress accounts for about 80% of all medical visits.

Intuitively, I knew the importance of joy as a therapy, though I had never researched it. It seems like common sense when you say that humor, laughter, and joy are good for your health. After all, the wisest man who ever lived, Solomon, said that a joyful heart is good medicine, but a crushed spirit dries up the bones. When I asked Angie when she last laughed, her eyes filled with tears, and she sobbed uncontrollably. Through her tears, she told me how she hadn't smiled, laughed, or had an ounce of joy for months. She described the perpetual darkness that filled her days and nights. She conveyed her sense of hopelessness. At that time, we were all coming out of the COVID pandemic and isolation, and when I asked that question, she could no longer hold back her pent-up emotions. I listened intently and to her surprise, I smiled. I curved my lips into an ear-to-ear grin, and initially she looked offended. She thought I was laughing at her. I continued smiling, and soon a smile emerged from Angie. She even chuckled. The power of joy or humor was unleashed by my smile. Joy is contagious.

Angie's smile in that moment can be explained through the fascinating concept of mirror neurons. These special brain cells allow us to observe and comprehend the actions, intentions, and motivations of others effortlessly and instantly. When we witness someone smiling, our mirror neurons activate, triggering the sensation associated with a smile.

Humor, Smiling, and Laughter

Smiles are most often associated with positive experiences such as joy, humor, and laughter. Although the words are frequently used interchangeably, they have different definitions. Humor is the tendency of experiences to provoke laughter and provide amusement. Laughter refers to the physical reaction characterized by a repetitive vocal sound and facial expressions that are somewhat unique to us. People often have a distinctive laugh. My wife often tells me that I have my dad's laugh. My dad had a knack for generally finding humor, and as a result laughter, in everyday situations. I remember his rambunctious laughter, whether he was watching a TV show, playing a card game, or seeing his kids act silly. My dad knew how to laugh and find joy in life. The practice of medicine at times can be joyless and sometimes necessitates manufacturing humor and laughter. Often, when I'm on call, after doing hospital rounds, and seeing seriously ill patients, I'll go back to my office to interpret cardiac studies. Dealing with so much sorrow and pain is difficult. The stress from these emotions can be potent. This is precisely when I manufacture something to laugh at. I turn on my streaming service du jour and listen to my favorite sitcom, movie, or comedian play in the background while reading studies. Sometimes it seems like magic how quickly my mood shifts. Listening to the same punchlines triggers a genuine deep laugh that always lifts my spirits, allowing me to carry on throughout my day.

When something funny happens, our brains signal to our facial muscles, telling them to move and create a smile. As we start to laugh, our breath becomes faster, and we take in more air. This makes our chest and belly move up and down. Then, when something is really funny, the vocal cords in our throat start to vibrate, making funny sounds that we hear as laughter.

Laughter can be experienced individually or as a group. We laugh when we recall a funny event, watch a comedy, or socialize. I stop, more times than I can count, and literally laugh out loud. My wife will ask me what I am laughing about, since I'm alone, and I'll tell her that I was just thinking about something that happened in the past. Although smiling and laughter can be faked, it ensues naturally from humor.

The History of Humor in Medicine

Humor, laughter, and joy can be traced back to the earliest of human origins. In the late 1800s, archaeologists discovered an ancient clay tablet in Iraq. This tablet, dating back 4,000 years to the early stages of writing, contained what is believed to be the world's oldest recorded bar joke. The joke, written in the ancient Sumerian language, goes like this: "A dog enters a bar and says, 'I cannot see anything. I'll open this one.'" Get it? Scholars certainly did not. Nor did the thousands of Twitter and Reddit users who responded to a viral post.

In the Bible, there is a remarkable story in Genesis about the birth of Isaac, which involves laughter. Abraham, who was 100 years old, and Sarah, who was 90 years old, were unable to have children for a long time. However, God blessed them with a son despite their old age. Sarah acknowledges that it is God who made this miracle happen, and she names her son Isaac, which means "laughter." Sarah believes that her story will bring laughter to others. People might laugh with her and find joy in her story, or perhaps some may even laugh at the idea of a woman as old as Sarah having a baby. However, regardless of how others react, Sarah is grateful to God for the laughter and happiness that Isaac brings into their lives.

There is also a history of humor in tragedy. Charlie Chaplin once said, "In order to truly laugh you need to be able to take your pain and play with it." This was a somber reference to the importance of transforming pain into joy through humor and laughter. I knew it was important for my patients to have joy in their lives, so I kept asking them when they last laughed. Of course, Angie was skeptical and asked, "Doc, is there any evidence that this is real medicine, or is this just fake stuff?" Her question jump started my deep exploration into laughter and joy. I wanted to find out how humor and laughter relate to health, wellness, and medicine. Let's look at the earlier quoted Bible verse Proverbs 17:22: **A joyful heart is good medicine**, but a broken spirit dries up the bones. This points us to the conclusion that people long ago understood that a joyful spirit has a positive therapeutic effect on us, while the absence of joy makes one ill.

The World Health Organization defines health as a state of complete physical, mental, and social well-being. Health is not merely the absence of disease and infirmity. When we talk about the joy of life, we refer to more than the absence of pain or sadness. Joy is the presence of humor and laughter.

Centuries ago, Indigenous North American nations like the Iroquois used clown-like performers to entertain and make the sick person laugh, believing that laughter had healing properties. This tradition of using humor in healing has influenced the use of healing clowns in modern healthcare settings. More recently in the 14th century, French surgeon Henri de Mondeville used humor to distract his patients from pain during surgery. De Mondeville believed it was important to keep his patients comfortable, cheerful, and hopeful. Current studies validate his work, revealing that humor and laughter modulates or changes the impression of pain. Mondeville based his book, *Cyrurgia*, on his experience with patients. He advised surgeons to regulate the patient's entire life. Basically, he advocated taking a holistic approach that included joy and happiness. He suggested allowing relatives and friends to visit the patient, and he advised joviality and joke telling. The famous 16th century German priest Martin Luther used humor to treat psychiatric disorders as a critical component of his counseling. He advised that depressed individuals should surround themselves with friends who could joke and make them laugh. Sixteenth century English scholar Robert Burton extended this practice by using humor to treat psychiatric disorders. In the 17th century, Herbert Spencer, who was a sociologist, used humor as a relaxation technique. And the 18th century? Both Immanuel Kant, a German philosopher, and William Battie, an English physician, used humor to treat illness.

My research told me I was on to something. Laughter has been prescribed for centuries to treat mental and physical problems.

What Happens to the Body When You Laugh?

Let's look to science to see how laughter affects the body. Science points out that laughter is exercise. Laughter relaxes the face muscles and improves respiration, and improved respiration increases blood flow. This results in a decrease of stress hormones and an increase in the body's main defenses. This cascade effect then alleviates pain and raises the pain threshold and increases our tolerance to pain. These changes enhance mental functioning.

Humor and Norman Cousins

The case of Norman Cousins provides a benchmark for arguing the efficacy of laughter and humor in health. Back in 1964, after a highly stressful trip to Russia, Cousins received a devastating diagnosis of ankylosing spondylitis, a degenerative disease that causes collagen breakdown and results in severe and persistent pain. His doctor warned him that he had only a few months to live, painting a grim picture of his future. But Cousins didn't give in to despair. Instead, he developed a compelling theory: If stress played a role in his illness, then cultivating positive emotions could potentially alleviate his suffering.

With the approval of his doctors, Cousins made a bold decision. He left the hospital and found refuge in a nearby hotel. There, he crafted a regimen for himself that involved consuming high doses of vitamin C and immersing himself in an uninterrupted flow of amusing films and other sources of laughter. Astonishingly, Cousins discovered that just ten minutes of hearty laughter granted him a remarkable two hours of relief from pain, surpassing even the effectiveness of morphine. Gradually, his condition started to improve, and he regained mobility in his limbs. Within six months, he found himself standing on his own feet again, and within two years, he was back at his full-time job at the *Saturday Review*. This astounding recovery left the scientific community bewildered and sparked numerous research projects on the subject.

Cousins's journey highlights the profound impact of laughter and humor on our overall well-being. He recognized that chronic stress elevates stress hormone levels, such as epinephrine and cortisol, which can increase the risk of cardiovascular and other diseases. In contrast, positive emotions have the potential to reduce the risk of stress-related disorders. Cousins understood that laughter acted as a natural anesthetic for his body, and it ultimately saved his life. He lived and thrived for an additional 15 years, exemplifying the psychobiological effects of laughter.

Continuing his exploration of the connection between human emotions and biochemistry, Cousins joined the staff at the University of California, Los Angeles (UCLA) in 1968. He dedicated himself to further research on the subject, firmly believing that sustained laughter and joy were key factors in resisting and combating illness. He frequently emphasized the link between negative emotions and negative physiological responses, while positive emotions, in his view, led to positive physiological outcomes. Cousins firmly believed that positive emotions were not only restorative but also contributed to building resilience within the body.

Since Cousins's case, multiple studies on laughter as a stress reducer and healing agent have been released. In 40 short years, laughter therapy spread throughout North America. Professor William Fry, M.D., of the Stanford University School of Medicine developed a theory of laughter therapy. He reached the same conclusion as Cousins: Humor and laughter actually produce natural pain killers. During laughter, pain killers, or endorphins, are released in the pituitary gland. The endorphins improve blood circulation and decrease stress.

The Importance of Humor

One laughter theory is called the Motion Creates Emotion Theory (MCET). The MCET postulates that the body does not know the difference between intentional or instinctual laughter. If the body doesn't know the difference—if the body reacts the same way to both stimuli—then we gain the same effects whether we *fake it 'till we make it* or laugh spontaneously. We can capture the positive benefits of spontaneous laughter without using humor and when there's nothing funny happening. We can smile and fake laughter even when we are in physical or emotional pain. It worked for Norman Cousins, and we now have science-backed evidence to prove it. Put daily smiles on your to-do list and notice how much better you feel.

The Impact of Humor and Laughter on Stress

In a recent study conducted in 2020, researchers aimed to understand how laughter influenced the experience of stressful events and the symptoms of stress. They focused on university students, who commonly face a multitude of stressors in their daily lives. The study examined the frequency and intensity of laughter and how these factors affected the participants' perception of stress.

To assess the impact of laughter, the researchers looked at its presence, frequency, and level of intensity. They wanted to determine whether a light chuckle, a deep belly laugh, or a knee-slapping uproar made a difference. Surprisingly, they discovered that the frequency of laughter during a stressful event was linked to a decrease in subsequent stress symptoms, such as heart palpitations and dry mouth. The more often the students laughed, the weaker the association between experiencing a stressful event and reporting stress-related symptoms became.

However, what's even more intriguing is that the intensity of laughter had no effect on this association. In other words, it didn't matter if the laughter was genuine or forced, or whether it was a boisterous laugh or a gentle chuckle. Both high-intensity and low-intensity laughter yielded similar beneficial effects in reducing stress symptoms following a stressful event.

Based on these findings, the authors of the study concluded that frequent laughter was associated with lower stress symptoms when confronted with stressful events. Surprisingly, the intensity of the laughter didn't play a significant role in this relationship. So, whether you find yourself faking it or just barely cracking a smile, both approaches can have the same positive impact on alleviating stress.

The Impact of Laughter on Stress Hormones

Laughter is a wonderful way to relieve stress and feel good. It has been studied for many years and has been found to have positive effects on our body and mind. Researchers have uncovered how laughter lowers stress through our hormones. In a landmark study conducted in 1989, scientists wanted to understand how laughter affects our stress response. They studied 10 healthy men, half of whom watched a funny video while the other half didn't. The researchers took their blood samples to measure different hormones related to stress. The results were fascinating. The group that watched the funny video had lower levels of stress hormones like cortisol and dopamine compared to the group that didn't watch the video. Laughter also reduced their levels of another stress hormone called epinephrine. The growth hormone in the laughter group initially increased and then decreased, while it remained the same in the other group. Other hormones didn't show significant changes.

So, laughing can actually make us feel less stressed and even affect our hormone levels. This is important because it shows that laughter can help our bodies cope with stress. This study was followed by more research, including one in 2003 that involved 33 healthy women. They watched funny videos, and the more they laughed, the less stressed they felt. Moreover, the women who laughed a lot had better immune system function.

This highlights the power of joy and laughter in improving our well-being and boosting our immune system. Something as simple as watching a comedy show for just 30 minutes can make us feel better. So, don't forget to laugh and find moments of joy in your life to take care of your mind and body.

The Benefits of Anticipating a Joyful Situation

The body eagerly responds to anticipation. I remember anticipating Christmas when I was young. I would count down the days. We had one Christmas that we affectionately labeled The Spiegel Christmas when my dad ordered our presents from the Spiegel catalog. There were boxes and boxes of gifts around the Christmas tree. My siblings and I could not wait to open the presents. Every time I went into the living room, my eyes would open wide, eager with anticipation. I was excited and happy. I wondered if I was going to get what I wanted. The emotions were exhilarating.

The body is like a kid before Christmas, because it anticipates what's going to occur and releases hormones in anticipation of an event. This reaction is well established as it relates to eating and blood insulin. When we smell food, our parasympathetic nervous system activates the digestive system. Remember, the parasympathetic system is the network of nerves that relaxes your body after periods of stress and hunger. It assists processes like digestion. When the parasympathetic nervous system smells food and anticipates eating, the parasympathetic nervous system triggers saliva production and increases insulin levels. Insulin tells the body to store blood sugar so the body can use the anticipated incoming nutrients. This hormonal activity makes us feel hungrier.

I remember going to hear the comedian Chris Tucker. I started chuckling before his performance just thinking of the way he said certain words or remembering lines from one of his movies. I laughed in anticipation of the upcoming fun time and the laughter that would ensue.

There was a study conducted to evaluate the proposed theory that the anticipation of laughter reduces stress hormones. The study looked at 16 healthy fasting men and studied their cortisol levels and catecholamine changes. When we are stressed, the hormones cortisol and catecholamine are released. Researchers assigned participants to a control group or an experimental group. The experimental group was the group that was anticipating a humorous event. Blood was drawn from participants in both groups prior to the event, four times during the event, and three times after the event. The blood levels of the experimental group revealed a decrease of cortisol, epinephrine, and the breakdown of dopamine. These three hormone levels continued to decrease throughout the event. The researchers suggested that just anticipating a positive event can decrease detrimental stress hormones. Hopefully, we will use studies like these to guide and motivate us to reduce our stress levels.

The Impact of Everyday Lifestyle Choices

There is growing evidence that our lifestyle choices—everything we do—impacts our health. This realization feeds into the health equation that health equals resiliency divided by stress. Everything we do adds to our resiliency or to our stress. When researchers began to look deeply into how our lifestyles impact our health, they found that everything has consequences. What we eat, when we eat, and how much we eat affects us. How much we exercise, whether we smoke or not, our alcohol consumption, where we live, the air we breathe, shift work, our social circles—all these behaviors and choices impact our DNA. Lifestyle choices do not affect DNA sequencing but they do impact the epigenome: chemical compounds that modify, or mark, genes in a way that tells them what to do, where to do it, and when to do it.

Epigenetic regulation, which occurs in our DNA, is the process of turning our DNA on and off. Epigenetic regulation occurs when certain environmental factors have an effect on the expression of certain genes. Our choices impact us all the way down to our basic physiological functioning. Our choices turn our propensity toward disease up or down. Our choices also affect our microbiome. Our microbiome, as you may remember, consists of the synergetic relationship between bacteria and human cells. From our mental health to our physical health, the microbiome can predict disease.

Now let's look at some of the research concerning lifestyle. Researchers used 20 non-smoking healthy men and women in their early 30s. Participants had normal blood pressure, cholesterol, and blood sugar. Researchers assessed their artery function and their brachial artery flow mediated dilatation reactivity after an overnight fast. The fast excluded activity, supplements, and alcohol. Participants then watched movies while lying down in a temperature-controlled room for about 30 minutes. They selected movies that would either increase stress or invoke laughter. Participants were to watch the movies to the point where they felt like they were being affected by the movie. They watched the 1998 movie *Saving Private Ryan* as the stressful movie and *Something About Mary* for its comic effect. Results showed that 14 out of 20 volunteers had a decreased brachial flow mediated dilatation after watching *Saving Private Ryan*. For the comedy, 19 out of 20 participants had increased vessel dilation. Obviously, those who watched the comedy had a healthier outcome. The flow media dilatation difference between the mental stress and after phases exceeded 50% in otherwise healthy men and women. This study shows that stress inhibits the healthy flow in our vessels. These results apply to other stressors such as emotional anger recall and solving math problems, which, too, have been evaluated for vessel response.

Research shows improvements in flow mediated dilatation after laughter. The same kind of improvement was previously observed after aerobic activity or statin therapy. Researchers hypothesize that stress impairs a process in the endothelium which results in damage to the endothelium. These well researched interviews led researchers to conclude that positive emotions, like laughter, have a beneficial effect on the lining of the vessels in the heart and that laughter can heal a broken heart.

The Impact of Laughter on Heart Disease

In 2001, researchers conducted a simple study to see if laughter, when studied in a large population, is associated with a reduction of coronary heart disease. In this study, researchers questioned 300 people about their anger and hostility, as well as how often they laughed in different situations. Researchers administered questionnaires that assessed anger and hostility or measured the propensity to laugh under different situations that occur in everyday life. The results showed that people with heart disease were less likely to experience laughter during daily activities, surprise situations, or social interactions compared to those without heart disease. Even after considering other factors like high cholesterol, high blood pressure, and diabetes, a strong connection was found between a sense of humor and a lower risk of heart disease. This means that the lower your humor, joy, and laughter, the higher your risk for coronary heart disease even after adjusting for other variables such as high cholesterol, high blood pressure, and diabetes. Conversely, the more you laugh, and the more joy in your life, the lower your risk of heart disease, and the more likely you are to cure a broken heart.

A 2013 gerontological evaluative survey conducted in Japan analyzed the data of nearly 21,000 participants. Participants were equally divided between men and women who were roughly 65 years old. The participants provided, by mail, data on their daily frequency of laughter and their weight, along with other cofactors such as where they lived, income, lifestyle, and whether they were diagnosed with cardiovascular disease, high blood pressure, high cholesterol, or depression. Even after taking out the impact of high cholesterol, high blood pressure, depression, and body mass index, the likelihood of a person who rarely or never laughed was nearly 21% higher for having heart disease than those who reported laughing daily. The risk for stroke was nearly 60% higher for those who never laughed compared to those who laughed every day. We might say that laughter is the key to life.

The Yamagata study prospectively investigated associations of daily frequency of laughter with mortality and cardiovascular disease in a community-based population. Researchers looked at 17,000 individuals who were approximately 40 years old. They were questioned during their annual checkup. Researchers looked at their self-reported frequency of laughter. Participants were grouped into three categories: those who laughed once per week, those who laughed once per month, and less than once per month. Researchers looked for associations between the frequency of laughter and the increase in all-cause mortality and cardiovascular disease. Results showed that all-cause death and cardiovascular disease was significantly higher in subjects with the low frequency of laughter. Once again researchers adjusted for age, gender, high blood pressure, smoking, and alcohol consumption. Results still showed all-cause mortality was significantly higher in subjects who laughed less than once per month compared to subjects who laughed more than once a week. A similar risk of cardiovascular events was higher in subjects who never laughed compared to those who laughed once or twice a month. These results should motivate us to find reasons to laugh, given that laughing is heart healthy.

Laughter as Therapy

I remember a friendly patient, a woman in her late 40s, from before the COVID pandemic. She had two young sons and a job with irregular hours that made it hard for her to visit the doctor regularly. Unfortunately, she had a heart attack, and I recommended cardiac rehabilitation. This program focuses on exercise, healthy eating, stress reduction, and adjusting medications as needed to reduce the chances of another heart attack and improve quality of life. However, her inflexible work hours made it impossible for her to attend. She missed important appointments, and I couldn't monitor her risk factors and medication. Sadly, after five months without seeing her, I learned she had another heart attack. This was a wake-up call for me because I realized I needed to find a way to help people who couldn't come to the office. So, I started using technology like phones, video calls, and remote examination tools to connect with patients. This led to the creation of a successful virtual cardiac rehabilitation program.

During this journey, I discovered an article that emphasized the importance of joy in life, particularly through humor and laughter. Researchers had integrated humor into a cardiac rehabilitation program as a way to reduce stress, which is crucial for heart health. They conducted a study with 48 diabetic patients who had recently experienced a heart attack. They split them into two groups: one received traditional cardiac rehab, and the other, the experimental group, added humor to their program. The humor group got to choose what made them laugh and spent 30 minutes daily enjoying it. After a year, they had fewer heart rhythm problems, lower blood pressure, and reduced stress hormones. They felt better, had fewer heart attacks, and used less nitroglycerin. The study showed that humor can decrease stress hormones and decrease the risk of more heart attacks. So, laughter can be a valuable part of heart attack recovery. Once again, we see that humor and laughter can positively impact our health and mend broken hearts.

The Benefits of Smiling

Angie was going through a tough time, feeling vulnerable and down, and that's when I encouraged her to put on a smile, even if it didn't feel genuine at first. I told her, "Sometimes, you've got to fake it until you make it. Try to smile, focus on the good things in your life, and let go of the past. Believe it or not, even a pretend smile can do you some good. There's research showing that when we avoid frowning, it can lead to lower stress levels and more happiness. Your heart can benefit whether you're genuinely smiling or just putting on a grin."

I mentioned a study conducted at the University of Cardiff in Wales during our conversation. They had 25 participants at a clinic in London, where some received Botox injections to their foreheads while others had different cosmetic treatments. Two weeks later, everyone answered a mood questionnaire. Surprisingly, the group with Botox injections reported feeling significantly less depressed, anxious, and irritable. However, it wasn't the Botox itself; the idea was that not being able to frown, due to the injections, reduced their stress. This relates to the concept of "facial feedback," which suggests that the muscles in your face can affect your emotions. So, people who couldn't frown because of Botox tended to be happier overall than those who could. Now, I'm not suggesting you go get Botox, but it just goes to show that even something as simple as your facial expression can impact your health.

You might be surprised to learn that researchers have named what we think of as a genuine smile. It's called a Duchenne smile. A Duchenne smile reaches your eyes. There's a sparkle. It's easy to spot a fake smile or an obligatory smile. When we encounter someone with a Duchenne smile, we usually smile back.

A study conducted in 2012 measured the effect of smiles on stress. The participants were divided into two groups. Researchers gave individuals two sets of stressful tasks. One group was told to keep a smile on their faces even during stressful tasks. Some participants were given chopsticks to hold between their teeth to mimic a smile to ensure they wouldn't frown. The heart rates among the smiling group were lower during the stressful events than the heart rates of the control group. The calmest hearts were found in the participants who had the distinct smile. The smile resulted in their heart rates being stable. The authors concluded that there is physiologic and psychological benefit from maintaining positive facial expressions during stress.

Neurobiologist Peggy Mason concludes, based on research, that smiling with your eyes and your mouth can lift your mood, calm you down, and help you forge connections with other people. You can mimic, create, or express a Duchenne smile. Just smile from ear to ear and eye to eye to intentionally influence your body and mind. Your smile can influence other people's actions through mirror neurons.

Why is it important to smile? Why is it wise to incorporate joy and happiness into our lives? Hopefully, I have provided enough information for you to answer this question, but perhaps to convince you further, let's explore some other compelling studies.

Researchers looked at the risk and impact of happiness as it relates to years of life lived among US adults. This is different from the other studies that we discussed, since this study worked with those who have similar customs and lifestyles to those who reside in the United States. Researchers used a general social survey and the national death index data set to formulate their findings. Research revealed that compared to very happy people, the risk of death is 6% higher for individuals who are only pretty happy and 14% higher amongst those who are not happy at all. There is nearly a 10% difference in the likelihood of the length of time you live based upon whether or not you incorporate humor, joy, or laughter into your daily life.

Incorporating Joy into My Daily Life

Angie was unclear as to how she could incorporate joy into her daily life, so I tried to provide a format. Again, I told her to use the smart approach. "You have to be specific, your goal must be measurable, achievable, relevant to our ultimate goal, and time based." Maybe you will choose a partner to whom you can be accountable. Maybe you will choose a rewards calendar and put a check for each day you smile at someone. Place a checkmark on your calendar for each day you watch a comedy or read a joke. Choose how many days, weeks, or months you will participate in your laughter or smile experiment. Make it long enough to create a habit of happiness. Science tells us it takes about 66 days to make a lifestyle change. The goal is not to break the chain of happiness or smiling habit for as long as your stated time frame. Make your goals sound. Be sure to consider your values and morals when choosing your actions.

What makes us smile or laugh? How can we fake it? Suggestions follow but remember to design your goals

personally. What is fun or funny for you?

- Choose a comedy over a horror movie. Studies support this choice. A comedy will help you borrow some joy even when your life is complicated and difficult. Watching someone else laugh is a fantastic way to fake it 'til you make it.

- Wear a smile when in pain. I remember hiring an energetic nurse. I was amazed at how everything he said sounded pleasant or happy. I remarked to him, "I need to learn from you. You have a calming and enjoyable countenance." "Doc," he replied. "Just smile when you speak." He nailed it. Smiling even changes one's tone. He wasn't aware of the research on smiling, but his life provided an example of how smiling affects oneself and others. A smile radiates positive energy, and that energy seeps inside and lifts our spirits and heals our bodies.

- Reflect and think of the happy times in your life. Savor the moments of joy every day.

- Smile at everyone you encounter.

- Actively sing. Participating in music-making has a positive impact on our brain chemicals, like dopamine and serotonin, which affect our mood. When we actively make music, whether by singing, playing an instrument, or creating electronic music, it can bring us closer to others by releasing oxytocin, a hormone that promotes connection. Singing together in a group helps us synchronize our breathing, promoting relaxation and reducing cortisol, which is known as "the stress hormone." Overall, making music is a great way to feel good and reduce stress.

- Greet yourself in the mirror at the start of the day with a smile and say, "I am going to smile today! Today I create more happiness in my life."

- Buy a joke book and read a joke a day or get free daily jokes by email.

We've learned that the higher your joy in life, the lower your stress, and the higher your joy in life, the better your health. Humor, joy, and laughter are essential to our health and an integral part of the road to better health.

CHAPTER 9

Conclusion

Your Want, Your Will, and Your Won't

W hat do you want? What are you willing to do to get what you want? What won't you do? Research led by social psychologist Roy Baumeister shows that willpower is like a muscle. But muscles tire. As you use your willpower muscle throughout the day, it weakens. Haven't you ever awakened in the morning with good intentions? "Today I will be positive and friendly. I will be kind to my children. I will not shout. I will start on that diet. I will exercise and eat wisely." But as the day moves along, you are barraged by stressors. It's the kids, the job, the traffic jam, the tiff with your partner, or the red light blinking in the car. It's too much. The cumulative stress erodes your willpower. Researchers estimate that adults make about 35,000 conscious and unconscious decisions every day. Even when it comes to the food we make, approximately 226.7 decisions are made each day according to researchers at Cornell University. By the end of the day, you are trying to emotionally survive. Your goals and emphatic intentions are left behind in the dust of daily duties. Your willpower muscle weakens as you make multiple complex decisions.

The power to transform requires three components of self-control. We need self-control more than willpower, but willpower is vital. Kelly McGonigal describes in her book *The Will Power Instinct* the need for the *will power, want power, and won't power*. Will power (What will you do to get to your goals?) is doing what you need to do even when you don't want to or feel like doing it. Will power says no to temptation. *Want power* is remembering what you really want when you face temptation. Won't power (What won't you do to get to your goals?) allows you to say no when you need to say no, and yes when you need to say yes. We want to change, but before we can change, we must lay a foundation. The most important aspect to change is our mental outlook. Our outlook is our foundation. Henry Ford said, "Whether you think you can, or you think you can't —you're right." This thought highlights the power of mindset. Our mindset matters. It counts in work, in relationships, and in health. Our perspective shapes how we feel, what we believe, and how we act. And most importantly, our outlook profoundly affects our health.

Studies have revealed that our mindset, or our expectations regarding healing, can have a profound impact on our bodies. These effects can be observed in various systems within our bodies, including the immune system, cardiovascular system, and neuroendocrine system. In simpler terms, our thoughts and beliefs about healing can actually influence the way our bodies function at a biological level. Often people become impatient or frustrated because what they desire doesn't happen overnight. They focus on the finish line and overlook the daily steps or habits needed for change. Aristotle said, "We are what we repeatedly do. Excellence, therefore, is not an act; it is a habit." Change is a process that takes time and is best accomplished one habit or step at a time. This slow methodological process is similar to the philosophical debate over the ship of Theseus. Theseus, for those who are not fans of Greek mythology, was a divine hero and founder of Athens. As a tribute to Theseus, after he rescued the children of Athens, his ship remained in the harbor and sailed once a year. After several centuries of maintenance, each plank of the Ship of Theseus was replaced. The philosophical question becomes, "Is it still the same ship now that all the parts were replaced?" It was still a ship, though the components all changed. Getting Self*ish* changes you and challenges you to transform your life one plank at a time. Getting Self*ish* challenges you to focus on the daily process. When we change our lives one plank at a time, we are still us, just as the ship was still a ship after all the parts were changed, but we will be healthier and happier. As we go through life, evolving and growing, change doesn't wipe away our identity. Instead, it uncovers and unveils new layers and dimensions of our true selves.

How Habits Form

"Bad habits are like a comfortable bed; easy to get into but hard to get out of."

Habits form when our actions become automatic, like taking the same route to work every day. Sometimes we develop habits without even trying, but we can also intentionally create or get rid of them to achieve our personal goals. We all have many habits, whether we realize it or not, that help us meet our needs more easily in daily life. However, because habits become deeply rooted in our brains, it can be tough to break a habit that causes more harm than good. If we understand how habits are formed, it can be useful in getting rid of old habits and replacing them with new ones.

Habits and the motivational triad are closely related. The motivational triad is a principle that attempts to understand why we do what we do. The principle is based on the concept that our brain is wired to seek pleasure, avoid pain, and conserve energy. These are the drivers that play a big role in forming habits. Seeking pleasure and avoiding pain are strong motivators for individuals to engage in certain behaviors repeatedly. For example, if someone finds pleasure in eating unhealthy foods (like chocolate cake or ice cream) due to the release of dopamine in the reward pathway of the limbic system, they may develop a habit of reaching for those foods whenever they want to experience pleasure. In other words, when we do something that brings us pleasure or rewards us, our brain releases a chemical called dopamine, which makes us feel good. This makes it more likely that we will repeat that behavior in the future.

Similarly, avoiding pain can also drive the formation of habits. For instance, if someone experiences anxiety or stress and finds that engaging in a particular behavior, such as smoking, shopping, or excessive alcohol consumption, temporarily alleviates those negative emotions, they may develop a habit of resorting to those behaviors whenever they want to avoid or reduce their discomfort.

Habits play a crucial role in the interplay between the motivational triad and the limbic system. Habits are automatic, repetitive behaviors that are often driven by the limbic system and are influenced by the motivational triad.

The limbic system is a part of our brain that deals with emotions, motivation, and memory. It helps us associate certain cues or triggers with pleasurable experiences. For example, if we always eat a snack while watching TV, the limbic system associates the TV with the pleasure of eating. This makes it harder to break the habit because our brains crave that reward.

The limbic system, particularly an area of the brain called the basal ganglia, is involved in habit formation and execution. When a behavior is consistently rewarded or associated with pleasure, the limbic system reinforces the neural connections related to that behavior, making it more automatic and habitual. This process is known as reinforcement learning.

The limbic system's involvement in habit formation and the influence of the motivational triad can create a feedback loop. Habits can reinforce the seeking pleasure and avoiding pain aspects of the motivational triad, as engaging in certain behaviors becomes automatic and rewarding. In turn, the limbic system further strengthens the neural connections related to those habits, making them more difficult to break.

Understanding the role of habits, the motivational triad, and the limbic system can be helpful in both developing positive habits and breaking negative ones. By consciously aligning our behaviors with the motivational triad, we can create habits that support our goals and well-being. Additionally, understanding the underlying mechanisms of habit formation can inform strategies for breaking unwanted habits by disrupting the reinforcement learning process in the limbic system.

Let's look at the Cue-Routine-Reward system. The cue-reward system is a fundamental process in the formation of habits, as it helps explain why certain behaviors become automatic and difficult to change. When behaviors are consistently linked with rewarding outcomes, our brains strengthen the connections between cues and those behaviors, making them more ingrained and habitual. This system harnesses the power of instincts to help us change our habits, stop habits, or develop new habits. The cue in Cue-Routine-Reward is the trigger that reminds the brain to do something. The cue is the prompt that kicks off the habit behavior. The cue usually falls into one of several categories. The cue can be triggered by a certain location, a place, a time, an emotional state, people around you, or your last action.

The Routine is the second aspect of the habit loop or creation of repeated behaviors. A routine can be something that you may or may not be aware of. As I began to reflect on my personal experience, I realized I have many unconscious routines. As my kids began to grow, one of the many traditions we set was family movie time. This evolved from simple home Veggie Tales videos to the full-blown movie theater experience on opening night of the latest blockbuster film. The experience was never complete unless there were snacks like a big bucket of popcorn. Over time, whether at home or at a movie theater, the mere suggestion of watching a movie became the cue and the routine was to reach for popcorn and snacks. In the example from my family, the cue of movie watching prompted the unconscious routine of eating popcorn.

The third aspect of the system is the reward. The reward refers to what the behavior gives you. How does it satisfy you? What is the reward? The reward will reinforce your routine and keep you stuck in your bad habit. For me, it's that crunch of popcorn. Maybe for you it is the smell, the taste, the mouth feel that gives you the reward. The cue, routine, reward concept of habit formation definitely is in play, but that is not all that is in play in habit formations like these. Many foods, like the movie theater popcorn, cookies, and candies, were constructed to heighten the reward process. These snacks all have something in common: crunch factor, vanishing calories, and a distinctive aroma that keep you craving more. Scientists have discovered that the audible sound from biting a food (crunch) triggers an individual perception of the food and increases desire. Researchers have also found that food that melts down quickly in the mouth tells your brain it's having no calories, and your brain gets fooled into thinking the calories have vanished, making you much more likely to keep eating before the brain sends you a signal that you've had enough. Investigators have previously demonstrated that the mere sight and smell of food can cause a release of dopamine, a neurotransmitter associated with motivation and pleasure.

When we want to break a habit, we have to identify the routine and figure out what the routine gives us so we can experiment with rewards that offer a similar experience. The theater popcorn gives me that crunch and satisfaction whether I'm hungry or not. Substituting movie popcorn for rice cakes or having air pop popcorn is one solution, but there may be others.

When you want to start a new behavior, such as working out four times a week, you might reward yourself with an enjoyable outing or a smoothie. Anticipating the reward can motivate you to act so you can get the reward.

Birds of a Feather – Our Secret Weapon

Why is the saying "Birds of a feather, flock together" important? My parents noticed how I picked up the habits of the groups or people I hung around. This is universal; we pick up the habits of those around us. Researchers have long studied the idea of "social contagion theory," which suggests that our friends' habits can influence our own, whether good or bad. The "social contagion theory," developed by Harvard professor Nicholas Christakis, suggests that our friends can influence our behaviors and habits. It means that bad habits like obesity, smoking, and unhappiness can spread through our social connections, even to friends of friends, up to three degrees of separation. In other words, the people we associate with can impact our choices and behaviors, and this can extend beyond just our immediate friends.

Research has also demonstrated that our friends can positively affect us. The people we socialize with or hang out with can become our secret weapon. They can help us achieve our goals. When you surround yourself with people with similar values and goals, you absorb the group components. We can use this human tendency to our advantage. We can tap into the motivation and support of people in our day-to-day lives. We can garner support from household members. They can influence our ability to follow through with our goals. If we live alone, don't spend much time with our families, or our families are not supportive of our goals, we can still get support. If you work outside the home and need outside support, look to your coworkers. Many of us spend 8 to 10 hours a day with our coworkers, which means we spend more than a third of our lives away from our families. In this case, our coworkers become our surrogate families. Choosing coworkers who have similar intentions to collaborate with can supercharge our growth. If you don't work outside the home, you can reach out to neighbors, church members, or our sports teammates. We do not need to gut it out by ourselves. Be creative, as Hellen Keller put it, "Alone we can do so little, together we can do so much." One inspiring example of this can be found in Daniel Zoughbie. Inspired by his grandmother's death from diabetes, he founded Microclinic International (MCI) to promote healthy behaviors through small peer groups. Their success in combating diabetes in other countries led them to try a similar approach in Bell County, Kentucky, where rates of obesity, diabetes, and high blood pressure are high. Participants formed close-knit groups to support each other in adopting healthier habits, and the results were impressive. By the end of the 40-week program, 95% of participants showed significant improvements in various health indicators. This success emphasizes the power of social connections in creating positive changes, no matter where we are in the world.

Planning

Planning is the most important first step in making comprehensive changes. The late British Lord Harold Samuel, the real estate tycoon, said, "There are three things that matter in property. Location. Location. Location." Similarly, I would say, "The three most important actions to take when changing a habit, or starting a new one, are to plan, plan, plan." This is the first key to succeeding in getting Self*ish*. When you plan, you eliminate the need to rely on your willpower. Planning is crucial, especially when you're too tired to make good decisions. Two essential components of planning are the implementation intention and premortem planning. The implementation intention is a plan that states that if X happens, then I will do Y. Premortem planning is a managerial strategy we can use to help us achieve our goals. This formula specifies an anticipated goal relevant to the situation. For example, a situation (X) arises, and you imagine possible solutions (Y) to mitigate the problem. Perhaps your goal is to eat healthily today, but you find yourself surrounded by fast food restaurants and you haven't had time to shop. The goal is to work backward to determine the potential solutions that can lead to your success. Too many lifestyle books highlight miraculous transformation stories where the caterpillar turns into the butterfly without obstacles, but that isn't real life. These fairytale stories often tap into our emotions. The stories focus on the goals, not the process, and often set us up for failure. Though not everything in our lives will go wrong, *some* things will. And things tend to go wrong at inopportune times. We must have contingency plans to circumvent failure in the face of setbacks.

A 2001 study examined people who wanted to exercise more. The participants were divided into three groups. The control group wrote down how often they exercised. The second group was provided with information on how to exercise. They attended lectures highlighting the benefits of exercise, and after this education, they recorded how often they exercised. The third group went a step further. In addition to getting information on exercise and attending lectures, they formulated a plan. They planned when, where, and how they would exercise over the following week. Each member completed the following sentence: "During the next week, I will partake in at least 20 minutes of vigorous exercise on such and such day at such and such time and in such and such place." Results found that the participants in groups one and two exercised 35% and 38% of the time. Their outcomes were approximately the same. The motivational lecture and reading didn't change the outcome. We can identify with this situation. How often have we listened to the same keynote speakers, attended numerous health conferences, watched the same kinds of documentaries, purchased more and more exercise equipment or books, yet have not seen the changes we desired? The results in the third group, the group that planned, were astounding. They exercised

91% of the time. This research discovered the participants' desires and turned them into action. These results remind us that if we want to make changes or achieve our goals, we need to plan, plan, plan. Success isn't so much dependent on your level of motivation; it depends on your plan. The plan, called implementation intention, supports one's goals by planning the when, where, and how to achieve our goal.

Let's look deeper at the process of premortem planning. The concept was developed by Gary Klein and published in the 2007 *Harvard Business Review*. Klein based the idea of premortem planning on the postmortem examination. The postmortem is an autopsy conducted after a person dies to determine the cause of death. Obviously, the postmortem doesn't help the person, because it is a retrospective action taken after death. At this point, nothing can save the person, but Klein's premortem starts before the challenge arises.

You can use premortem planning prior to taking action. What do you plan to do? What is your commitment? Eat healthy foods? Keep a gratitude or forgiveness journal? Meditate? Practice mindfulness? Look at your goal and imagine that it has failed. Think of all the possible scenarios of failure. Let's take the prior example of wanting to eat healthy foods.

Here's how the plan could fail:

- I'm hungry, and there are junk food snacks available everywhere at work.

- I'm attending a potluck dinner with all my favorite unhealthy foods and desserts.

- I'm hungry, and the only restaurants around are fast food restaurants.

- I go grocery shopping when hungry and buy things that aren't healthy.

- I lose my willpower when I'm tired.

After brainstorming all the possible dilemmas, it's time to devise a plan.

Here are some possible solutions:

- Carry an apple and nuts with me so I can have a healthy snack to tide me over while I go to the grocery store. I don't shop when I am hungry.

- Have healthy food or meals delivered to my home.

- Plan when I can shop for healthy foods. Put it on my calendar as a goal. When I shop, I stock up for the future.

- Start a meal calendar and plan each meal in advance.

- Take healthy snacks to the office so I won't be tempted to eat poorly when I am hungry or tired.

- Have healthy frozen foods at home so I can still eat well even when I am too exhausted to cook.

- Keep cut vegetables like celery and carrots available in the refrigerator.

I discovered several reasons for failing at eating healthy foods. I was inclined to eat unhealthy processed snack foods when my energy was low. This occurred when I had not eaten nutrient-rich calories. When I got home after work and walked through a snack-filled kitchen, I couldn't resist. I solved this by bringing more food to work, having healthy food to eat on my trip home, and entering my home through another entrance.

What Happened to Angie?

I wish I could tell you that Angie lived happily ever after, that she was completely transformed by the principles of Selfish. But this is a real-life story. Angie's journey had its successes and challenges. First, she denied that she ever had a problem. She believed that everyone else had the problem! Theoretical model psychologists describe this stage as the pre-contemplative stage.

In this stage, individuals do not recognize that they have a problem, or they recognize the problem but they're not ready to change. It's easier to recognize others' problems than to see our own problems. We naively recognize health issues in others while thinking these issues will never happen to us.

Angie needed that proverbial shoulder to cry on, and I gave her one. She, like we all do, wanted someone to understand her difficulties. My first step was to acknowledge and validate Angie's pain. I empathized with her. I offered my compassion. Her pain was real. Her children grew up and left home, she went through a divorce, and her mother died without her getting a chance to say goodbye to her or the family. Those stressful life circumstances were real, and I needed to confirm her difficulties, but I couldn't stop there. I knew that life is 10% what happens and 90% how we respond to those events. Our responses to challenges depend on our resiliency and our ability to bounce back. And our resiliency is linked to our health. As you well know, health equals resiliency divided by stress. The greater our resiliency, the better our health. The higher our resiliency, the more we are able to heal a broken heart and overcome stress. Getting Self*ish* will not prevent what happens, but it will optimize that 90% area where we have choice.

Angie finally realized that she had more choices than she had imagined and that building her resiliency would strengthen her ability to act and react in healthier ways. I watched Angie move through the stages of change. She eventually entered the contemplative stage and realized that she had a problem. Maybe her response was the problem, though, at the time, she wasn't always willing and ready to change her way of thinking. During this stage, people often weigh the pros and cons of changing their behaviors. Angie eventually moved to the preparation and determination stage as she readied herself for change. She committed. This commitment was part of her motivation to change. She entered the next phase of change—taking action, or doing the work. After a period of time, she entered the maintenance phase. She maintained healthful behaviors; not all the Self*ish* pillars simultaneously, but she took time for spirituality, exercise, love, forgiveness, and gratitude. She ate whole food—fiber-rich, plant-based foods. She developed intimacy through positive relationships, developed better sleep habits, and found a renewed joy in life. Since her life was not a fairytale, there were times when she relapsed. When Angie fell short of her plans, or fell off her self-constructed program, I encouraged her to renew her efforts. And she did, on numerous occasions. We can identify with this, because going back to our old habits is a human tendency. We abandon our plans. I encourage you, as I encouraged Angie, "Don't give up hope. It's okay to fall down but get back up again." Getting back up should be a part of your plan.

It's time for you to construct your plan to create new habits and release the unhealthy ones.

1. Start with a signed contract to yourself. Write out what you want to do, what you will do, and what you won't do. Sign it. This is your commitment to yourself.

2. Adopt a rewards calendar. Mark each day that you perform the desired behavior with an X or a star sticker. Put an X or sticker on the day that you meditate, pray, or offer gratitude. Mark each day that you eat healthy foods such as fruits, vegetables, whole grains, nuts, or seeds. Mark the days you exercise.

3. Find an accountability partner or group. You can meet virtually or in person; the important aspect is to find someone who holds you accountable for achieving your goals.

4. Choose small achievable goals. If you plan to run a marathon, commit to running 100 yards a day the first week. Find the time of day that works best for you. Over time, increase the distance you run. You want to create a habit. Your success revolves around setting achievable goals.

It's like the ship Theseus: You want to build your body and increase your resiliency one plank at a time. Remember the concept of making small changes, small achievable goals? A daily 1% change makes you 37 times better over the course of a year. If you start out with $100 at the beginning of the year and increase that amount 1% every day, at the end of the year, you'll have $3,778.34. That's 37.8 times more than what you had at the beginning of the year.

5. Enjoy the process. Focus on the process, not the finish line. This allows you to be present so you can experience that joy of life and feel as if you are living life on purpose.

Sel*fish*

Is getting Sel*fish* unique? The acronym SELFISH is unique, but the guiding principles behind Sel*fish* have been known and utilized since the beginning of time. Hopefully, after reading this book, you understand clearly that getting Sel*fish* isn't about individual promotion. Getting Sel*fish* is about becoming the best version of yourself so that you can live a life of purpose. Although I have promoted the individual components of Sel*fish* to my patients for years, the principles did not take shape until I read this quote from one of the greatest NBA players, Michael Jordan: "To be successful you have to be selfish, or else you never achieve..."

Achieving your goals is different from getting Sel*fish*. *Being selfish* is egocentric. Being selfish means being self-centered, lacking the ability to understand any perspective other than one's own. *Getting* Sel*fish* is about transformation and building the needed resiliency to bolster your mental and physical health. This resiliency allows you to live a life of service to your community and family. The Sel*fish* principle is different from those offered in other traditional wellness books because it takes a holistic view of the health journey. The Sel*fish* principle recognizes that health is the sum total of life experiences and emphasizes the power of incremental habit changes. These small steps result in keystone habits. Keystone habits are the foundation for transformation. These beneficial habits unintentionally carry over into other aspects of our lives.

Spirituality, exercise, and love in action are essential pillars of the principles of Sel*fish*. They are keystone habits. These keystone habits allow for the successful transformation of the central pillars of health and food. Each principle, individually and collectively, reduces stress and heals the broken heart. Adopting these foundational principles allows for easier transitioning to a fiber rich, whole food plant-based diet—a diet that relieves nutritional stress.

The journey toward getting Sel*fish* incorporates the second half of the previously mentioned Michael Jordan quote. "And once you get to your highest level, then you have to be unselfish. Stay reachable. Stay in touch. Don't isolate." The latter pillars of the Sel*fish* principle address the value of intimacy in relationships and the importance of being part of a community or tribe. But having a tribe alone is not enough. We need the right people in our tribe. Think about my parents saying, "Birds of a feather flock together." This points out the necessity to find a like-minded community. We need friends who have the same goals and aspirations as ourselves. Those who journey before us offer support and serve as role models. The power of modeling received from people on a similar journey has the potential to propel us to achieve success. They pave the way for us. Others, who have the same struggles as us, remind us that we are not alone and inspire us to keep traveling that bumpy road to success and transformation.

The Sel*fish* principle continues by including a frequently overlooked component to achieving our goals—sleep. We discussed the role of sleep in setting the table for success along with the power of focus and clarity of mind. The Sel*fish* principle concludes with incorporating humor, laughter, or joy into our lives. The goal isn't just to achieve our end results, it is to have fun and to engage in humor and laughter along the way.

Humor is an essential form of human existence.

I hope you use my personal story and research to support your health journey. Medical professionals can only take you so far. The Self*ish* principles can work in your life, and you deserve a robust and healthy life. I can't say good luck, because it will take more than luck to make changes in your life, so I leave you with these words: "It's time to get Self*ish!*"

Connect with our community at www.DrBatiste.com.

———————

REFERENCES

Stress

Jacobs, D.R. New England Journal of Medicine. 2022; 386: 1877-88.

Radfar, A. European Heart Journal. 2021; 42: 1898-1908.

Sher, L. American Journal Physiology Heart Circulation Physiology. 2020; 319: H488-H506.

Salleh, M.R. Malaysian Journal of Medical Sciences. Vol. 15, No. 4. October 2008. pp. 9-18.

Spikes, T. JAMA Network Open. 2022; 5(2): e220331.

Lazzarino, A. Journal American College of Cardiology. Vol. 62, (18). 2013.

Tawakol, A. Journal American College of Cardiology 2019; 73: 3243-55.

Assad, J. Clinical Medicine Insights: Cardiology. 2022; 16: 11795468211065782.

Lyon, A.R. Journal American College of Cardiology 2021; 77: 902-21.

Mariotti, A. Future Science OA. 2015; 1(3): FSO23.

Tawakol, A. Lancet. 2017; 389: 834-45.

Richardson, S. The American Journal of Cardiology. 2012; 110: 1711-1716.

Hinterdobler, J. European Heart Journal. Volume 42, Issue 39, 14 October 2021, pp. 4077–4088.

Zannas, A.S. Genome Biology. 2015; 16: 266.

Dimsdale, J.E. Journal American College of Cardiology. 2008; 51:

1237-46.

Framke, E. European Heart Journal. Vol. 41, pp. 1164-1178.

Kubota, Y. JAMA Internal Medicine. 2017; 177(8): 1165-1172.

Vaccarino, V. JAMA. 2021; 326(18): 1818-1828.

Mostofsky, E. Circulation. 2012; 125: 491-496.

Cohen, S. New England Journal of Medicine. 1991; 325: 606-12.

Jacobs Jr., D.R. New England Journal of Medicine. 2022; 386: 1877-1888.

Harvanek, Z.M. Translational Psychiatry. 2021; 11: 601.

Keys, J.D. JAMA Internal Medicine. 2022; 182(4): 445-448.

Mefford, M.T., et al. Journal of the American Heart Association. 2023; 12: e028332.

Mefford, M.T., et al. Proceedings of the National Academy of Sciences of the United States of America. 2020; doi:10.1073/pnas.2012096117.

Spiritual

Schneider, R.H. American Journal of Preventive Cardiology, 8, 100279. doi:10.1016/j.ajpc.2021.100279.

Friedfeld, P. (2022, September 1). Mindfulness and meditation can improve overall health for people with diabetes. Healio Endocrinology. https://www.healio. com/news/endocrinology/20220901/mindfulness-and-meditation-can-improve-overall-health-for-people-with-diabetes.

Carrière, K. Obesity Reviews, 19(2), 164-177.

Brewer, L.P.C. Journal of the American Heart Association. 2022; 11:e024974.

Medlock, M., et al. McLean Hospital spirituality and mental health consultation service: A novel approach to integrated treatment. 2022. Presented at American Psychiatric Association Annual Meeting; May 20-24, 2017; San Diego.

Keefe, R. Mental Health, Religion & Culture. 2016; 19:7, 722-733.

Levine, G. Journal of the American Heart Association. 2017; 6:e002218.

Kotchen, J. American Journal of Preventative Cardiology 2021; Oct 4; 8: 100279.

Schneider, R.H. Ethnicity & Disease. 2019; Oct 17;29(4):577-586.

McClintock, C.H. Current Behavioral Neuroscience Reports. 2019; Rep. 6, 253–262.

Ferguson, J.K Pastoral Psychology. 2010; 59; 305-329.

Beldling, J. Journal of Religious Health. 2010; 49: 179-187.

Tusche, A. Journal of Neuroscience. 2016; April 27, 36(17): 4719-4732.

Karadas, C., et al. Abstract 20343. Presented at ESC Acute Cardiovascular Care Congress; March 13-14, 2021 (virtual meeting).

Ference, B.A. Journal American College of Cardiology. 2018; Sep., 72(12): 1382–1396.

Rozanski, A. Journal American College of Cardiology 2014; July, 64(1): 100–110.

Levine, G.N. Circulation. 2021; 143: e763–e783 doi:10.1161/ClR.0000000000000947.

Rao, A. European Journal of Preventative Cardiology. 2020; March, 27(5): 478- 489.

Exercise

Allen, J. Progress in Molecular Biology and Translational Science. 2015 July 31; 135:337-354.

Aengevaeren, V.L. Circulation. 2020; 141:1338–1350.

Chodzko-Zajko. Medicine and Science in Sports and Exercise. 2009 Dec.;41(12):2128-35.

Malhotra, P. Acta Scientific Medical Sciences. 2019; 3(5):132-137.

McCleod, J. Frontiers in Physiology. 2019 June 6; 10:645.

Pollock, M.L. Circulation. 2000; 101:828–833.

Liu, Y. Medicine and Science in Sports and Exercise. 2019 Mar; 51(3):499–508.

Anderson Sports, E. Medicine and Health Science. 2019 Dec; 1(1):3–10.

Anderson, E. International Journal of Behavioral Nutrition and Physical Activity. 2021 Sep. 15; 18(1):123.

Winzer, E.B. Journal of the American Heart Association. 2018; 7:e007725.

Stamatakis, E. Journal of the American College of Cardiology. 2019 April; 73(16):2062–2072.

Piercy, K.L. Journal of the American Medical Association. 2018; 320(19):2020- 2028.

Bruning, R.S. Progress in Cardiovascular Diseases. 2015 Mar-Apr; 57(5):443– 453.

Gao, J. Journal of Cardiovascular Translational Research. 2022 June; 15(3):604- 620.

Cook, C.M. Journal of the American College of Cardiology. 2018 Aug.; 72(9):970– 983.

Zhang, H. Journal of the American College of Cardiology. 2018 Oct.; 72(14):1622–1639.

Eijsvogels, T.M.H. Journal of the American College of Cardiology.

2016 Jan.; 67(3):316–329.

Martinez, M.W. Journal of the American College of Cardiology. 2021 Oct.; 78(14):1453–1470.

Paluch, A.E. The Lancet Public Health. 2022 March; 7(3):e219-e228.

Inoue, K. JAMA Network Open. 2023; 6(3):e235174.

Berry, J.D. Journal of the American College of Cardiology. 2011 April; 57(15):1604–1610.

Lavie, C.J. Circulation Research. 2015; 117:207-219.

Hambrecht, R. New England Journal of Medicine. 2000; 342:454-460.

Long, X. Journal of Applied Physiology (1985). 2010 June; 108(6):1766–1774.

Pearce, M. JAMA Psychiatry. 2022; 79(6):550-559.

Stubbs, B. The Lancet Psychiatry. 2018; 5:736-746.

Nystoriak, M.A. Frontiers in Cardiovascular Medicine. 2018; 5:135.

Di Francescomarino, S. Sports Medicine. 2009; 39(10):797-812.

Laufs, U. Arteriosclerosis, Thrombosis, and Vascular Biology. 2005; 25:809–814.

da Silveira, M.P. Journal of Sport and Health Science. 2019 May; 8(3):201–217.

Schmidt-Trucksäss, A. Atherosclerosis. 2021 Sep.; 333:85-86.

Silva, J.K.T.N.F. Atherosclerosis. 2021 Sep.; 333:91-99.

LaCroix, A.Z. Biomed Central (BMC) Public Health. 2017 Feb. 14; 17(1):192.

Love

Waltman, M - Psychology and Health 24.1 (2009): 11-27.

Han, S - Social Science & Medicine 201 (2018): 120-126.

Lawton, R. - Journal of Happiness Studies 22.2 (2021): 599-624.

Harris, A. - Journal of Health Psychology 10.6 (2005): 739-752.

Baker, B. - American Journal of Hypertension 12.2 (1999): 227-230.

Holt-Lunstad, J - Annals of behavioral medicine 35.2 (2008): 239-244.

Acevedo, B - Social cognitive and affective neuroscience 7.2 (2012): 145-159.

Ricciardi, E. - Frontiers in human neuroscience 7 (2013): 48075.

Wang, P. Frontiers in Neuroscience 13 (2019): 454.

Thibonnier, M Endocrinology 140.3 (1999): 1301-1309.

Davis, D. Journal of counseling psychology 62.2 (2015): 329.

Sesan, R. Routledge, 2008. 235-248.

Horstman, Judith. The Scientific American book of love, sex and the brain: the neuroscience of how, when, why and who we love. John Wiley & Sons, 2011.

Marazziti, D. Recent Advances in NGF and Related Molecules: The Continuum of the NGF "Saga" (2021): 249-254.

Van T. Social Psychological and Personality Science 6.1 (2015): 47-55.

Long, K. BMC psychology 8 (2020): 1-11.

Akhtar, S. Trauma, Violence, & Abuse 19.1 (2018): 107-122.

da Silva, S. The Journal of Positive Psychology 12.4 (2017): 362-372.

Friedberg, J. International Journal of Behavioral Medicine 16

(2009): 205-211

Cousin, L. The Journal of Positive Psychology 16.3 (2021): 348-355.

Carpenter, T Personality and Individual Differences 98 (2016): 53-61.

Berretz, G, Public Library of Science (PLOS ONE). 17(5), e0266887.

Fisher, Helen. Why we love: The nature and chemistry of romantic love. Macmillan, 2004.

Chida, J Journal American College of Cardiology. 2009. 53(11), 936–946.

Cousin, L. The Journal of Positive Psychology, 16(3), 348–355.

Toussaint, L Journal of Health Psychology 21.6 (2016): 1004-1014.

Seawell, A. Psychology & Health 29.4 (2014): 375-389.

Han, S. Social Science & Medicine 201 (2018): 120-126.

Baker, B. American Journal of Hypertension 12.2 (1999): 227-230.

Harris, A. Journal of Health Psychology 10.6 (2005): 739-752.

Food

Safford, M - Circulation 143.3 (2021): 244-253.

Mendy, V International journal of environmental research and public health 15.9 (2018): 2016.

Freeman, A. Journal of the American College of Cardiology 69.9 (2017): 1172- 1187.

Jardim, T.V. The Public Library of Science (PLOS) Medicine. 2019; 16(12): e1002981.

Mendy, V. International journal of environmental research and public health 15.9 (2018): 2016.

Vogel, R.A. The American journal of cardiology 79.3 (1997): 350-354.

Gupta, K. Nutrition reviews 80.3 (2022): 400-427.

Kim, H. Journal of the American Heart Association 8.16 (2019): e01286

Quek, J. Frontiers in cardiovascular medicine 8 (2021): 756810.

Argyridou, S. The Journal of nutrition 151.7 (2021): 1844-1853.

Wang, F. Journal of the American Heart Association 4.10 (2015): e002408.

Honerlaw, J.P. Clinical nutrition 39.4 (2020): 1203-1208.

Pacheco, L.S. Journal of the American Heart Association 9.10 (2020): e014883.

Siegel, K.R. JAMA internal medicine 176.8 (2016): 1124-1132.

Baynham, R. Nutrients 13.4 (2021): 1103.

Jenkins, D.J.A. New England Journal of Medicine 384.14 (2021): 1312-1322

Rauber, F. Nutrition, Metabolism and Cardiovascular Diseases 25.1 (2015): 116- 122.

Huang, J. JAMA internal medicine 180.9 (2020): 1173-1184.

Edwards, L. Journal of exposure science & environmental epidemiology 32.3 (2022): 366-373.

Hall, K.D. Nature medicine 27.2 (2021): 344-353.

Byrd, D.A. The Journal of nutrition 149.12 (2019): 2206-2218.

Jackson, M.K. Antioxidants. 2023; 12(4): 946.

Millan-Orge, M. Scientific Reports 11.1 (2021): 20301.

Caitlin, A. Applied Physiology, Nutrition, and Metabolism 40.7

(2015): 711-715.

Freeman, A Journal of the American College of Cardiology 72.5 (2018): 553-568.

Keogh, J. Arteriosclerosis, thrombosis, and vascular biology 25.6 (2005): 1274-1279.

Dod, Harvinder S. The American journal of cardiology 105.3 (2010): 362-367.

PJL Ong Lancet. 1999 Dec.; 354(9196): 2134.

Nicholls, S.J. Journal of the American College of Cardiology 48.4 (2006): 715-720.

Good, S. Arteriosclerosis, thrombosis, and vascular biology 37.6 (2017): 1250-1260.

Weiss, E.P. The American journal of clinical nutrition 88.1 (2008): 51-57.

Boegehold, M.A. Journal of vascular research 50.6 (2013): 458-467.

Rudolph, T.K. The American journal of clinical nutrition 86.2 (2007): 334-340.

Keogh, J. B. Arteriosclerosis, Thrombosis, and Vascular Biology. 25(6), 1274-1279.

Chen, H. BMC medicine 21.1 (2023): 307.

Ding, K The American Journal of Clinical Nutrition 118.1 (2023): 201-208.

Wang, A. Proceedings of the National Academy of Sciences 120.18 (2023): e2221097120.

Mente, A. European heart journal 44.28 (2023): 2560-2579.

Wang, L. Journal of the American Heart Association 12.15 (2023): e029215.

Belardo, D. American Journal of Preventive Cardiology 10 (2022): 100323.

Leung, C.W. JAMA Network Open 6.6 (2023): e2321375-e2321375.

Sellem, L. BMJ (Clinical research ed.), 382, e076058.

Bonaccio, M. European Heart Journal 43.3 (2022): 213-224.

Glenn, A.J. Journal of the American Heart Association 10.16 (2021): e021515.

Medawar, E. Translational psychiatry 9.1 (2019): 1-17.

Akbaraly, T.N. The British Journal of Psychiatry 195.5 (2009): 408-413.

Beezhold, B.L. Nutrition journal 9 (2010): 1-7.

Lucus, M. Brain, behavior, and immunity 36 (2014): 46-53.53.

Agarawal, U. American Journal of Health Promotion 29.4 (2015): 245-254.

Satija, A. Journal of the American college of cardiology 70.4 (2017): 411-422.

Chazelas, E. European Journal of Public Health 30.Supplement 5 (2020): ckaa165-573.

Juul, F. Journal of the American College of Cardiology 77.12 (2021): 1520-1531.

Sun, Y. JCI insight 2.19 (2017).

Hui, S. European journal of nutrition 58 (2019): 2779-2787.

Koutentakis, M. Journal of cardiovascular development and disease 10.3 (2023): 94.

Iatan, I., Author2, A. A., & Author3, B. B. (2023). Featured Clinical Re- search II. Paper presented at the American College of Cardiology Scientific Session, March 4-6, 2023, New Orleans (hybrid meeting).

Li, S. Journal of the American Heart Association 3.5 (2014): e001169. Glabska, D. Nutrients. 2020 Jan.; 12(1): 115.

Bagatini, S. European Journal of Nutrition 61.6 (2022): 2929-2938.

Bagatini, S. Frontiers in Nutrition 9 (2022): 928.

Intimacy

Hawkley, L.C. Nature Reviews Disease Primers 8.1 (2022): 22.

Cené, C.W. Journal of the American Heart Association. 2022; 11:e026493.

Vallée, A. International Journal of Environmental Research and Public Health 20.4 (2023): 2869.

Elovainio, M. Lancet Public Health. 2023; 8: e109–18

Goodlin, S.J. Heart Failure 11.3 (2023): 345-346.

Valtorta, N.K. Heart. 2016;102:1009-1016.

Holcomb, Sarah. "What Trees Teach Us About Community and Crisis." Christianity Today, 2021, https://www.christianitytoday.com/better-samaritan/2021/april/what-trees-teach-us-about-community-and-crisis.html.

Reblin, M. Current opinion in psychiatry 21.2 (2008): 201-205.

Baker, B. American Journal of Hypertension 12.2 (1999): 227-230.

Hoang, P. JAMA network open 5.2 (2022): e2146461-e2146461

Grant, Richard. "Do Trees Talk To Each Other?" Smithsonian Magazine, www.smithsonianmag.com/science-nature/the-whisper- ing-trees-180968084/.

Egolf, B. American journal of public health 82.8 (1992):

1089-1092.

Holt-Lunstad, J. Public Library of Science (PLoS) medicine 7.7 (2010): e1000316.

Hostinar, C.E. Current opinion in psychology 5 (2015): 90-95.

Ozbay, F. Psychiatry (edgmont) 4.5 (2007): 35.

Wang, X. International journal of mental health systems 8 (2014): 1-5.

Kaveladze, B. International Journal of Social Psychiatry 68.2 (2022): 253-263.

Don, B. P. Social Psychological and Personality Science. 15(3), 288-298.

Pressman, S.D. Health Psychology 24.3 (2005): 297.

Gallagher, S. Brain, Behavior, and Immunity 103 (2022): 179-185.

Valtorta, N.K. Heart July 2016. Vol. 102 No. 13.

Hawkley, L.C. Psychology and aging, 21(1), 152-164.

Luo, Y. Social Science & Medicine. 74(6), 907-914.

Xia, N. Antioxidants & Redox Signaling. 2018 28:9, 837-851.

Kearns, A. Psychology, health & medicine 20.3 (2015): 332-344.

Sleep

Kohler, M. American journal of respiratory and critical care medicine 178.9 (2008): 984-988.

Hruska, B. Psychology & Health. 35:1, 1-15.

Hybschmann, J. Sleep Medicine Reviews. 59 (2021). 101456.

Calvin, A. Journal of the American Heart Association 3.6 (2014): e001143.

Aggarwal, B. Journal of the American Heart Association 7.12

(2018): e008590.

Domínguez, F. Journal of the American College of Cardiology 73.2 (2019): 134-144.

Petrovic, D. Cardiovascular research 116.8 (2020): 1514-1524.

Simon, E.B. Nature human behaviour 4.1 (2020): 100-110.

Konishi, T. Heart Vessels. 34, 1266–1279 (2019).

Münzel, T. Hypertension. 2021; 78:1841-1843.

Liew, S.C. Sleep Medicine. 77 (2021) 192-204.

Kingsbury, J.H. Current cardiovascular risk reports 7 (2013): 387-394.

Cowie, M.R. Journal of the American College of Cardiology 78.6 (2021): 608-624.

Li, X. Journal of the American College of Cardiology 78.12 (2021): 1197-1207.

Cowie, M.R. Journal of the American College of Cardiology 78.6 (2021): 608-624.

Covassin, N. Journal of the American College of Cardiology 79.13 (2022): 1254- 1265.

Huang, T. Journal of the American College of Cardiology 75.9 (2020): 991-999

Daghlas, I. Journal of the American College of Cardiology 74.10 (2019): 1304-1314.

Full, K.M. Journal of the American Heart Association. 2023; 12:e027361.

Nikbakhtian, S. European Heart Journal - Digital Health. Vol. 2, Issue 4, December 2021; Pages 658–666.

Makarem, N. Journal of the American Heart Association. 2022; 11:e025252.

Charles, L.E. International journal of emergency mental health 13.4 (2011): 229.

Chen, R. Sleep Health. 2023 April; 9(2): 211–217.

Hirotsu, C. Sleep Science 8.3 (2015): 143-152.

Thompson, K.I. Frontiers in behavioral neuroscience 16 (2022): 945661.

Salfi, F. Nature and Science of Sleep. 2020; 12:309-324.

Acheson, A. Physiology & behavior 91.5 (2007): 579-587

Harrison, Y. Organizational behavior and human decision processes 78.2 (1999): 128-145.

Morales, J. International Journal of Psychophysiology 96.3 (2015): 169-175.

Papatriantafyllou, E. Nutrients. 2022 April; 14(8): 1549.

Humor

Miller, M. Medical hypotheses 73.5 (2009): 636-639.

Sugawara, J. The American journal of cardiology 106.6 (2010): 856-859.

Bennett, M.P. Alternative therapies in health and medicine, 9(2), 38–45.

Tan, S.A. Advances in mind-body medicine, 22(3-4), 8–12.

Hayashi, K. Journal of epidemiology, 26(10), 546–552.

Ikeda, S. Journal of epidemiology, 31(2), 125–131.

Eraydin, C. Advances in integrative medicine, 9(3), 173–179.

van der Wal, C.N. Social science & medicine (1982), 232, 473–488.

Miller, M. Heart. 2006 Feb.; 92(2): 261–262.

Noureldein, M.H. Diabetes research and clinical practice, 135, 111–119.

Vlachopoulos, C. Psychosomatic Medicine 71(4):p 446-453, May 2009.

Yoshikawa, Y. Nursing open, 6(1), 93–99.

Tamada, Y. Journal of epidemiology, 26(10), 546–552.

Savage, B.M. Advances in physiology education, 41(3), 341–347.

Sakurada, K. Journal of epidemiology, 30(4), 188–193.

Kramer, C.K. The Public Library of Science (PLoS) One 2023 May 23;18(5):e0286260.

Ikeda, S. Journal of epidemiology, 31(2), 125–131.

Enyeji, A.M. International journal of environmental research and public health, 20(9), 5713.

Louie, D. American journal of lifestyle medicine, 10(4), 262–267.

Lewis, M. Scientific reports, 8(1), 14720.

Mora-Ripoll, R. Complementary therapies in medicine, 19(3), 170–177.

Jang, K.S. International journal of environmental research and public health, 19(16), 10191.

Laughter Is Good For Your Heart, According To A New University Of Maryland Medical Center Study." ScienceDaily. ScienceDaily, 17 November 2000. <www.sciencedaily.com/releases/2000/11/001116080726.htm>.

Books

McGonigal, K. (2012). The Willpower Instinct: How Self-Control Works, Why It Matters, And What You Can Do to Get More Of It.

Duhigg, Charles. The Power of Habit. Random House Books, 2013.

Ratey, J. J. Spark. Little, Brown & Company. 2013.

Esselstyn, Caldwell B. Prevent and Reverse Heart Disease: The Revolutionary, Scientifically Proven, Nutrition-based Cure. New York, Avery, 2007.

Klein, Gary. https://hbr.org/2007/09/performing-a-project-premortem.

Ruiz, D. M. The Four Agreements. Amber-Allen Publishing. 2001.

Walker, M. Why We Sleep. Penguin Books. 2018.

Sapolsky, R. M. Why Zebras Don't Get Ulcers: A Guide to Stress, Stress Related Diseases, And Coping. New York, W.H. Freeman. 1994.

Lisle, Douglas J., Alan Goldhamer. The Pleasure Trap: Mastering the Hidden Force That Undermines Health & Happiness. Healthy Living Publications.

Chef, A.J. The Secrets to Ultimate Weight Loss.

ABOUT THE AUTHOR

Dr. Columbus D. Batiste

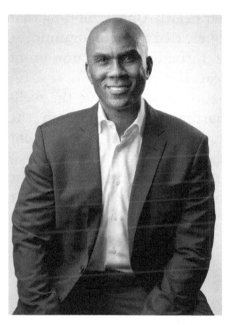

COLUMBUS D. BATISTE, MD, FACC, FSCAI is a double board-certified interventional cardiologist and assistant clinical professor at the University of California Riverside School of Medicine. From 2008 until 2020, he served as Chief of Cardiology. Dr. Batiste currently serves as the Regional Medical Director of Home-Based Cardiac Rehab and as Chair of the Regional Cardiac Quality Committee for the Southern California Permanente Medical Group.

Over the years, Dr. Batiste has been recognized for his work in the community and abroad by multiple organizations. In 2010, Dr. Batiste sought to break the cycle of prescriptions and procedures as the sole management of chronic disease and began promoting a long-term solution for his patients through nutrition, stress reduction, and exercise. As a result, in 2011, Dr. Batiste established the Integrative Cardiovascular Disease Program (based at Kaiser Permanente). This program aims to prevent the reoccurrence of major adverse cardiac events in patients who were diagnosed with a cardiovascular disease by focusing on lifestyle modification.

In 2016, Dr. Batiste led a group that collaborated with Samsung Technologies and developed a virtual cardiac rehabilitation program utilizing a Samsung wearable. Since its launch, the program, which applies the principles of the Selfish lifestyle, has treated nearly 10,000 patients. Dr. Batiste's mission is to share information so that "each one can teach one" about the benefits of plant-based nutrition, daily exercise, stress reduction, and therefore, provide everyone with the opportunity to take control of their health. Understanding that the health of an individual is uniquely tied to their community, Dr. Batiste collaborated on the formation of a non-profit organization called the Healthy Heart Nation.

The mission of Healthy Heart Nation is to improve the well-being of the community by narrowing disparities in the social determinants of health including education, employment opportunities and access to affordable healthcare services.

For more information about Dr. Batiste's initiatives, or to invite him to speak at your next event, please visit www.DrBatiste.com.